SECRETS *from the* OPERATING ROOM

SECRETS *from the* OPERATING ROOM

My Experiences, Observations, and Reflections as a Surgical Salesman

CURTIS M. CHAUDOIN

iUniverse, Inc.
Bloomington

SECRETS FROM THE OPERATING ROOM
My Experiences, Observations, and Reflections as a Surgical Salesman

iUniverse books may be ordered through booksellers or by contacting:

iUniverse
1663 Liberty Drive
Bloomington, IN 47403
www.iuniverse.com
1-800-Authors (1-800-288-4677)

ISBN: 978-1-4759-9166-6 (sc)
ISBN: 978-1-4759-9167-3 (hc)
ISBN: 978-1-4759-9168-0 (e)

Library of Congress Control Number: 2013908955

Printed in the United States of America

iUniverse rev. date: 6/18/2013

Contents

Preface
What I Want to Accomplish

For the past thirty-seven years, I worked in the most incredibly complex, fascinating, intriguing, and, sometimes, lurid world imaginable. It is a world that provided me with a lifetime of pleasure and frustration. It is a world that taught me humility and sobered me to what reality is. That world is the operating room.

During my career as a surgical salesman, I received extensive training and education that qualified me to work in the OR and assist in surgical procedures. I am not only certified to work in the OR. I am also certified to teach continuing education courses to OR nurses and technicians on a variety of surgical issues. Completion of these courses is required by OR nurses and technicians to maintain a valid license.

In the course of my years of surgical experience, I have gained invaluable knowledge about the surgical field. It is a field that is vitally important and pertinent to all of us. Why is it important? Every year, one out of every ten people will need to have a surgical procedure. The majority of those needing surgery know nothing about the operating room or surgery. And they will not have the information that is essential to making an educated decision about their entire surgical process.

Through this book, I attempt to contribute objective information and suggestions to help ensure that process has a rewarding outcome. I also have aspirations of reducing the anxiety that many surgical candidates feel about their medical condition due to their lack of surgical understanding and knowledge.

There have been many changes in the humanitarian mission of hospitals; the role of surgical corporations, whose instruments and equipment are used in the operating room; and the surgeon/patient relationship in the OR. I will give my opinion of how these changes affect the delivery of surgical care and of the problems associated with surgical corporations, and I will offer you a glimpse of what really occurs during a surgical procedure.

There are also personal reasons for writing this book. First, I wanted to do something that I had promised to do. That was to write a book about my experiences in surgery. Through the years, I told many operating room stories to friends and relatives at parties and functions. Each time that I would relate an experience, someone would say, "You should write a book on your experiences." So I am living up to that promise.

Writing a book has been an interesting challenge for me. Sitting and collecting your thoughts, trying to remember specific situations, and putting them into words on paper is an arduous task. Although I have my college degree in journalism, I have not worked in the journalistic arena since my time spent as a reporter and editor for the *University Daily Kansan* newspaper.

The foremost reward for writing this book is a feeling of personal satisfaction and achievement. Logically and methodically compiling ideas, memories, and words into a rhythmic body of work demands volumes and hours of thinking. It is a hate-love relationship. You hate the demands and frustrations of the work; you love the feeling of accomplishment when a successful day of writing is done.

It has been a refreshing turn back in time to retrace my path in life and see it through a more seasoned and mature prism. And to revisit those experiences required that I make a pledge to myself. I pledged to do the best that I could in objectively relating and remembering those events and experiences, without prejudice.

There is no doubt in my mind that this book will be viewed with mixed opinions and thoughts. That is okay. I have thick skin. You need thick skin to work in the operating room. I am quite confident and self-assured about everything that I have related. You also need confidence to work in the operating room. There will be naysayers who decry what I have to say. To those, I say that you are either ill-informed or have a vested interest in the surgical arena and profit from it.

I am satisfied with my book. It has given me peace of

heart and mind to write about an industry that I love and admire. My intentions are honest and honorable. I had no desire to make any disparaging remarks about any individual. I merely wanted to share my thoughts and feelings about an industry that few people know and understand.

I am very indebted to all of the true nurses and surgeons who, through our patient-care relationships, have made my life better and meaningful. They are very special people. I have fond memories and reflections of their dedication to health care, the tenderness that they show to their patients, and the manner in which they respected my devotion to serving.

Introduction
About Health Care

One of the more important issues in life is your personal health. Whether there is a caring, morally responsible and efficient health-care system in the United States should not even be a question. But after spending a lifetime working in health care, and specifically in surgery, there are many questions resounding in my mind. Are hospitals still devoted to humanitarian issues? Are corporate and individual profits more important than delivering affordable health-care services? Are surgeons more concerned about their personal issues than the health-care issues of their patients? Why are there increasing numbers of surgical mistakes each year?

Every year in the United States there are over thirty-four million surgical procedures performed. An ever-growing number of these procedures are performed in outpatient surgical settings. Questions have arisen about the quality of the surgical services provided in outpatient facilities compared to that in hospitals. The cost of my surgery may be less in an outpatient facility. But is there reason for concern about potential increased infection rates in outpatient facilities?

The number of reported surgical mishaps every year totals over four thousand. However, the number of actual surgical mishaps is estimated to be much higher because many surgical mistakes go unreported. By law, hospitals are required to report all surgical mishaps. How is it that so many could go unreported?

The surgical corporations that manufacture the instruments used in your procedure find themselves in a faltering situation. They use less-than-ethical means to persuade hospitals and surgeons to purchase their products. They rush instruments to market that fail during surgery, and in some instances these failures cause the loss of life. When will restrictions and legislation be enacted to ensure a more honest and safer environment for surgical patients?

How well do you know your surgeon? Have you researched your surgeon to find out if there is any pending litigation for surgical malpractice against him/her? Or are you using this surgeon because someone, with no medical knowledge, said that he/she was really good?

I have years of practical knowledge about the operating room and the secretive world of surgery. In this book, I offer suggestions and observations to help improve the state and outcome of your patient care. I present my opinions of hospitals, nurses, and surgeons. I believe that by increasing your awareness, you will be truly empowered to capture more control of your prospective surgical situation.

Also, I have chronicled my life as a surgical salesman. I share my personal experiences in several surgical procedures and medical situations to bring a human touch to the people in the OR. After all, there are many dedicated people in the OR with whom I have worked and fostered special relationships.

Chapter 1
The Life and Views of a Surgical Salesman

An Overview

After graduating from high school, I enrolled at the University of Kansas. I studied journalism and English. In 1971, I graduated with a bachelor of science in journalism. I was ready for the business world and all the exciting opportunities that were soon to be mine. At least, that was my perspective as an immature college graduate.

I will never forget a conversation that I had with my father at a party after college graduation. During the conversation, he said that there are four kinds of people in the business world. There are liars, whores, pimps, and thieves. And that they will do anything for money, power, and sex. He stated that if you are able to find a good, honest businessperson as a mentor, you will be a blessed person and enjoy your work. If not, your life will be a living hell. With that, he further emphasized that it is more important for whom you work rather than where.

As a very young man, I did not really understand that those words were pearls of wisdom. I was eager to capture the world. But I was too naïve to understand the world that I was about to enter, and how difficult that world would be. Now, after forty years in the business world, mostly in health care, I realize how brilliant my father was. I understand how true those words of wisdom really are.

Since 1975, I have been employed as an OR surgical salesman. During that time, I have worked for several different surgical companies. Besides the OR, I have worked in every procedural area in the hospital, including obstetrics, cardiac catheterization lab, GI lab, and the emergency room.

In my sales career, I have sold sterilization products and sterilizers, antiseptics and disinfectants, surgical scrub solutions, surgical drapes, surgical gowns, ECG electrodes, wound care dressings, surgical instruments, and surgical equipment. I have conducted hundreds of regular product in-services and lectured hundreds of CEU educational programs for OR nursing staffs. I have worked in and assisted in thousands of surgical procedures. And I have witnessed every kind of operation that can be performed, including an SRS. That is sex reassignment surgery, or a sex change procedure.

My ability to gain access into the surgical sales field

was a stroke of luck. Years ago, most companies that manufactured and sold surgical devices required that candidates have prior surgical sales experience before they would hire you. I had never worked in the medical field. I had no prior surgical sales experience. If you do not have surgical or even medical sales experience and cannot be hired, how do you get surgical sales experience so that you will be hired?

I was employed with one of the larger and more successful consumer product companies in the world. They manufacture and sell a variety of cleaning products to retail, institutional, and industrial consumers. I worked as a sales representative in their institutional division. The company wanted to start a surgical division, and I was asked to join. I was one of five salespeople, out of over thirty thousand employees, selected to start and operate this new division. It sounded exciting, and I accepted the offer. Heck, it was a nice increase in salary. And I believed that it would be a more prestigious position. Who would not want to have an increase in pay and advancement in position in the business world?

I received my first surgical training at a world-renowned university hospital in a large southern state. The training was conducted by the nurse educator for the hospital operating room. She was extremely experienced and savvy. She was very professional and took her nursing responsibility seriously.

Most OR nurses are very serious about their profession. They are very dedicated to and feel very passionate about patient care. My nurse educator was an ardent member of the AORN, or Association of periOperative Registered Nurses.[1] The AORN is an association that is very important to all OR nurses.[2] It is this organization that strives to improve patient care in the OR and actively works to maintain and improve safety standards.[3] There are chapters in every city or county area across the United States.

My first round of training lasted for three weeks. There were many topics and subjects to learn. We were taught the proper attire in the OR and how it should be worn; patient privacy issues; OR sterile fields; movement in and out of the OR; conduct in the OR suite; principles regarding asepsis, infection control, and safety; and fire risks. We were not allowed in any working OR, to actively view any surgical procedures, until after the first full week of training. There was a lot to see and absorb. There would be many more training courses in the months and years ahead.

My first day working in the operating room and viewing surgery was quite an overwhelming experience. I did not become nervous, ill, or feel faint. That is common for first-timers in surgery. It was the incredible array of procedures that I witnessed. The first procedure that I observed was a disarticulation below the right knee. It is also known as an amputation. It was slightly shocking. The second case that I monitored was an abdominal hysterectomy. Not as riveting as an amputation, but unnerving. It was the third procedure that shocked me beyond belief!

A teenage man was brought into the OR to have back surgery. It was a trauma case. He was involved in a car accident and arrived at the hospital by ambulance. He was immediately brought to the OR from the emergency room. The OR team took him from the ER stretcher, placed him on the surgical table, and began prepping him for surgery. Within minutes, he went into cardiac arrest. Immediately, the OR team began CPR and went for the crash cart. The mood in the OR quickly changed from relaxed and congenial to emergency mode. Loud voices, direct mandates, and quick actions prevailed. The circulating nurse told me to immediately leave the room. I quickly responded to her mandate and went to the OR nurses' lounge.

Approximately one hour later, she came to the lounge and told me that the young man had expired. She could see that I was quite shaken. She was very kind as she explained to me why I had to leave the OR and the appropriate protocol under those circumstances. She also taught me a valuable lesson that day. She said not to take anything that you see or hear in the OR personally. She said that the yelling and shouting that transpires during any OR situation is not personal—it is situational.

I went back to my hotel room that night emotionally drained and physically exhausted. I wondered if this was a job that I wanted to continue. I made a promise to myself to stick it out. I did not want to quit and wonder later if I had made a mistake. And I remembered the advice that was given to me by that OR circulating nurse. It helped to lessen my anxiety. I have never forgotten that advice or my first day in the OR.

I held a sales position with my first surgical company for four years. It was quite a learning experience and provided me entrance into an amazing selling society. However, I was ready to move on to another company. I did not enjoy the management by intimidation and fear philosophy that the company practiced. I hoped to find a company that subscribed to a different philosophy and stay in the surgical field. I loved the medical environment and working in surgery.

I quickly found another job through a recruiting firm. It was with a company in the surgical field. And, as I would learn, that management team treated employees with respect and integrity. I also found the business mentor that my father discussed with me years before. For the next twenty years, my business life would be a wonderful learning and growing experience with my mentor.

I enjoyed my new employer and my new sales position. The company was well established in its surgical niche, and it manufactured the highest quality products. It was the world leader in its field in the surgical industry. My business success was more than I could ever have envisioned. I relished waking up every morning and going to work.

David, the gentleman who hired me, was just that. He was a gentleman. I never heard David say a negative word about anyone. He treated everyone with a unique sense of respect and dignity. He led by example with every conversation, presentation, and interaction that he performed. For me, a young man finding his way in the business world, David was the perfect person to emulate. I could learn the proper and ethical way that business should be conducted.

More than once David proved to me that he was a man of genuine character. I remember a sales promotion that he was conducting with the sales force. Most companies do these promotions to make selling fun and allow the salespeople to earn some extra cash. There also are bragging rights associated with winning these promotions. Salespeople are very competitive. Don't let anyone convince you otherwise.

I won the sales promotion by making a huge sale to one of my university hospitals. The order was so large that it could not be filled by my company. And to make the problem even worse, the entire line of product that I sold was placed on a recall. No product to sell or ship, with any company, means no commissions for the salesperson.

I received a phone call from David. He congratulated me on the large sale and winning the promotion. He said that he had some bad news and some good news. He wanted to know which I wanted to hear first. I said the bad news. He said that the company would not be able to pay me any commissions because of the product recall. I said that I was disappointed; however, I understood. I asked him the good news. He said that the good news was that *he* would pay me the commissions.

I almost fell over. He was going to pay me several thousand dollars in commissions out of his own pocket. I told him that he did not have to do that. He said that he did. He said that when he hired me, I became part of his business family. He said that the product recall and the company's inability to fill the order was not my fault. He emphasized that I made the sale and that I deserved to be paid. After that act of kindness and generosity, I would do anything for him.

David and I successfully worked for that company for ten years. Sadly, the business world changes periodically. David saw that his time was up with our company and that it was time for him to move ahead. When he announced that he was leaving, I told him that I wanted to go with him. He said not to worry; he would call me. In fact, out of fifty salespeople in our division, all fifty wanted to go with him. No one knew where that would be, but it did not matter. We would have followed him anywhere.

David was not out of work for any length of time. He accepted a position as national sales manager with a small but growing surgical company. He called one day to offer me a sales position. I said yes without hesitation. That quickly, the world was right again.

Joining a new company and selling different types of surgical products meant more surgical and product training. The next series of training was not conducted in the OR. It was held in classrooms with a surgical training company. This training session was titled, "Codes of Conduct and Safety in Patient Care Settings."

Seminar topics included: patient rights and safety (HIPPA), role definition/codes of conduct, pathogens and blood-borne viruses, infection prevention, standard precautions, principles of asepsis, hazard protection, and fire safety.[4]

For another ten years I prospered, learned, and grew from David's example. Unfortunately, he had to retire early for medical reasons. Suddenly, the man who taught me a lifetime of ethical business professionalism would no longer be there.

I could never thank David enough for the lessons that I learned from him—and not just from a business perspective. He taught me life lessons. He taught me to be honest and humble in everything that I do in life. The last time that I spoke with him, I said thank you and good-bye. It was a wonderful conversation, although it was one of the sadder days of my life. I have not spoken with him for several years. I hope that he is doing well.

I stayed with that company for another thirteen years. There were several management changes during that time. The managers came, failed, took their options, and left. It happened repeatedly. The company was floundering and doing nothing to improve the working environment. Business was not fun anymore. The same old management philosophy of intimidation and fear kept appearing. I realized that the greatest obstacle that I had in performing my job and being successful was my own company. That was a sad awakening.

The one constant that kept me interested in work was

the operating room. It was like an addictive drug. With the operating room came excitement and fascination. It made you feel that you were participating in something meaningful. It required continuous training. I was constantly studying and learning about new surgical products, anatomy involved in specific procedures, and the step-by-step performance of the surgeon during those procedures. I was tested on products, technical specifications, and how and why instruments were used. It was never-ending. I loved it. It helped keep me going.

The operating room is a world unto itself. It is a world behind double doors. You will easily recognize where the operating room is. There is usually a sign that says, Stop! Do Not Enter, OR Personnel Only. It is a secretive and cloistered world that most people enter only when they have a surgical procedure performed. Most people know or understand very little about that world.

The secretive nature of the OR is intentional. The people who work in the OR follow a strict code of silence. You are not supposed to speak about procedures or patients outside of the OR suite. There is never to be conversation relating to any surgical procedure in elevators, hallways, waiting rooms, or dining areas. There could be a relative or friend of a surgical patient within ear range. Overheard conversations about patients may be a violation of their privacy rights and could be fuel for a lawsuit.

This manner of conduct is understood by every hospital employee from the housekeeping staff to nurses and medical students. During my first week of surgical training, I was in the cafeteria eating lunch. Sitting at the table next to me was a group of first-year medical students. They were talking and laughing about some of their patient cases. One of the head nurses from the OR happened to be walking by and heard their conversation. She instructed them to follow her. Ten minutes later the group returned. There was not a smile on any of their faces. Not one of them said a word. I can only imagine what was said to them in private.

I believe that the majority of people who are going to have surgery do very little research about their situation. They know very few facts about their hospital, the OR suite, the OR nursing staff, anesthesia, or their recommended surgical procedure. But most astounding to me, they know nothing about the attending surgeon who is about to invade their body! I cannot imagine committing yourself to surgery without doing extensive research on everything and everyone involved in the process. If you do no research as a patient, you will assume the worst and anxiously await your doom.

No one looks forward to being admitted to the hospital. And the thought of having to undergo a surgical procedure conjures up the worst fears and anxiety. Those fears and anxiety are understandable. It is natural to have a fear of anything that is unknown. We have heard horror stories of mistakes that occur in surgery, and we can visualize one happening to us. However, if you take the time to research and educate yourself about the surgical world, you will lessen your worries and fears. An educated patient is a confident and relaxed patient.

There is no average day in the OR. Each day is a day of miracles and tragedies, joy and sadness, success and failure. Many thousands of surgical procedures are performed every day in the United States and across the world. The procedural specialty fields include general, neurosurgery, orthopedic, vascular, urology, gynecology, plastics, thoracic, and obstetrics. Within each specialty comes new advanced techniques and instrumentation.

The rate of technique change in the surgical field occurs at a staggering rate. What was the standard practice six months ago is now outdated and passé. New instrumentation and modified technique are the constant norms.

The vast majority of surgical procedures performed run smoothly and have successful outcomes. And the reason for the high success rate is due to the knowledge, training, expertise, and professionalism of the OR team. Each member has spent years in training to achieve a license or certification in a specialty field. And each member spends many hours in continuing education courses, in-services, and seminars. This is a requirement to maintain a valid and current license or registration certificate.

There are times when procedures go terribly wrong. Sadly, even to the point of death. When you observe these tragedies, you agonize. Your body and mind are numb. Your mind searches for answers why. Sometimes the answers are clinically understandable. Sometimes they make no sense. Regardless, you have an ocean of feelings for the patient and the family. You also sympathize with the OR team.

All working people have stress in their lives. We all want to be successful and do the best job possible. We care about our work. It is impossible to end the workday and not bring the emotions and stresses home with you. I think that is human nature.

It is the same in the surgical world, with one exception. In the surgical world, every day you are dealing with people's health and their lives. I have the utmost respect for people in the armed forces, policemen and firemen, and nurses and doctors. They are special people for what they do and what they have to see. They possess a unique quality that enables them to combine mental toughness and character with nurturing care and a compassionate touch. I hold them all in the highest esteem. I feel blessed and honored to have been able to work and learn in that type of world.

Chapter 1 Endnotes:

1. AORN, Association of periOperative Registered Nurses, accessed December 5, 2012, http://www.aorn.com.
2. Ibid.
3. "Who We Are," AORN, accessed December 5, 2012, http://www.aorn.com/About_AORN/Who_We_Are.aspx.
4. "Excellence in Continuing Healthcare Education," Pfiedler Enterprises, accessed December 5, 2012, http://www.pfiedlerenterprises.com/about-us.

Chapter 2
Surgical Corporations

Profits and Risks

There are hundreds of surgical corporations in the United States. They differ in whether they manufacture products, distribute them, or do both. They also differ in where their products are manufactured, assembled, and packaged. The production and assemblage of surgical products in foreign countries has always been an area of contention with me. No other country in the world has the watchful eye that the United States has when it comes to product control and regulation. Do you want to have surgery with products made under the regulations of Mexico and China, or those made in the United States?

Regardless of how these companies manufacture, assemble, or distribute products, they have several commonalities. They want to make as much money as possible in the shortest amount of time, and they do not care how they do it or at whose expense. This may sound greedy, uncaring, and unethical. It is, and that is the surgical business.

I have serious reservations about surgical products made outside the United States. I have been in the operating room when sterile products were opened, and a foreign object—a fly, a roach, or a piece of hair—was found inside the package. This has occurred countless times. In the majority of these instances, the products were manufactured, assembled, and/or packaged in a foreign country. Why does this repeatedly happen to such a high degree?

Surgical products made, assembled, or packaged in Mexico, China, and other foreign countries cost the surgical corporation a pittance of what it would cost to be made in the United States. However, I believe that there is a difference in the quality of the surgical products made by dysfunctional, illiterate workers in a third-world nation and those made by skilled technical tradesmen in America.

I believe in the free-market enterprise system that we attempt or allude to in the United States. I do not, however, agree to the use of unethical and inferior production means in coordinating that system. Remember, it has been said that the business world is ripe with liars, whores, pimps, and thieves. The surgical industry and, in particular, surgical corporations employ some of the more egregious.

All corporations need profits to exist. This is true whether it is the medical, retail, institutional, or industrial market. Profits are needed for corporations to pay employees, grow and expand, and make more money for investors. But there also needs to be an ethical analysis of where a company may reduce production costs without sacrificing product quality and safety. This would be healthy and good for all parties involved. This should be the normal part of the free-market system too.

There is another questionable side to the surgical industry that disturbs me. It is quite common for companies to pay for breakfasts, lunches, and dinners in hospitals and surgeons' offices in order to present new instruments and equipment or to introduce new, advanced pharmaceuticals. I will admit that some hospitals have changed their rules and regulations. A growing number of hospitals will not allow companies to bring in anything that might be considered gratuitous. They are concerned about conflicts of interest.

I am completely in favor of looking at whether purchasing products from a company is influenced by the free benefits that medical personnel receive on a regular basis. After all, giving people something for free makes them feel obligated to you. Some of the surgical companies are now adopting the same approach and attitude, particularly the smaller companies. They cannot afford to spend the huge amounts of money that the large corporations do.

How rampant is the abuse of free breakfasts, lunches, dinners, and vacation seminars to buy business from hospitals, surgeons, and nurses? It is off the charts.

I spoke with a sales representative that works for a pharmaceutical company. This drug company is a worldwide organization. It employs thousands of sales people who call on doctors' offices and leave samples of different drugs. The sales representative told me that his company mandates that each salesperson spend at least $5,000 every month on lunches for surgeons' offices. The company monitors his expenses each month to verify his spending. He said that he must also do regular dinners, seminars, and lectures with groups of surgeons each month. That amount spent is more than twice his lunch expense. This is spending from just one salesperson in one pharmaceutical company. All of the pharmaceutical companies do it. They must, in order to compete. Surgical companies must perform and involve themselves in this type of behavior also.

Many surgeons will not make appointments with salespeople in the hospital or the OR to see new instruments or discuss new clinical technology. They want to see salespeople in their office. Often, the surgeon's office will not allow the medical salespeople to see the surgeon until they buy lunch for the entire office. You are informed of this when you try to make an appointment.

A regular day for the surgical instrument salesperson includes presenting instruments to surgeons. It is the only way that the surgeon can see an instrument and make an informed decision about evaluating in a clinical procedure. So if you have a new instrument that you want a surgeon to use, you are forced to buy lunch.

I was attempting to sell a new technological advancement to a group of orthopedic surgeons. This group was large and performed most of the orthopedic procedures in a particular hospital. I tried to see a few of the more influential ones in the OR between cases. They would not see me. These surgeons had an office next to the hospital. I decided to visit their offices and try to either talk to any of them between patients or make an appointment to demonstrate my wares.

I entered the office and introduced myself to the receptionist. I asked her if any of the surgeons were available to discuss new orthopedic instrumentation. She said that the doctors would only see salespeople if they did a luncheon for the office. My company had a pretty strict policy on lunches. If the total was less than one hundred dollars, I could do it if the surgeons would agree to evaluate the instrument in a procedure. If the surgeons would not evaluate, I would have a lot of explaining to do about why I did the lunch. I asked how many people were in the office. She said 150 office personnel, including the surgeons. I was in disbelief. A luncheon like that would cost over $2,000. I said no, thanked her, and left.

This is only one incident. But this story repeats itself with salespeople from every surgical instrument company in every surgeon's office every day. It is part of the avarice and greed that infests the surgical industry. It is reminiscent of a selfish gimme attitude.

The introduction of new surgical instruments by surgical companies is a key concern of mine. Companies are constantly racing to find new and improved surgical technologies and instruments to obtain a vital competitive edge. The best advantage for a company is to have an instrument or technology that nobody else has. This will allow the company to dictate pricing. One new, exclusive instrument may initiate tens of millions of dollars in profit. These new, advanced technology surgical instruments are expensive to buy. Some disposable, single-use instruments may cost a hospital thousands of dollars. And several of them may be needed and used in each procedure.

The federal government does have a process that surgical companies must follow to bring a new instrument to the market for sale. The process does take time, and there are strict guidelines. But I believe that the process and guidelines need to be more stringent. There needs to be more testing of instruments on cadavers and in animal labs before instruments are approved for use on humans in the operating room.

I have seen too many tragic surgeries where instruments have malfunctioned, broken, or fallen apart inside of a patient and caused serious organ damage and surgical complications. Each year, the number of reported surgical instrument malfunction cases is in the thousands. Tragically, some of these cases end in the death of the patient. By requiring more proof of an instrument's integrity before it is allowed for use on a human, could not the incidence of patient injury and death be drastically reduced?

In their haste to sell more and introduce new instruments to the industry at a faster pace, many surgical companies have adopted selling strategies and employment practices that are counterproductive and may be dangerous to patients.

All salespeople understand and accept the idea of quotas. It is the way by which employees are judged for merit, salary, and regular commissions. In years past, salespeople were given yearly quotas with quarterly benchmarks. If the quarterly benchmarks were attained, there were usually bonuses included. At the end of the year, based on your percent to quota achievement, you would know if you still had a job. It was customary, each year, to have only a 10 to 15 percent change in the sales positions. That included employees being terminated and those leaving on their own. This was healthy for the company. And it helped to ensure that the company employed a majority of experienced and knowledgeable salespeople.

Today, many surgical companies base the employment of their salespeople on a monthly or bimonthly basis. If the salespeople do not hit their monthly quota, they are put on probation. If they do not hit their quota the next month, they are terminated. This can be costly for the company if they are regularly firing and hiring so many employees. It has been reported that some surgical companies have 60 percent termination rates every year. And it is not uncommon for these companies to have an inside employment recruiter to reduce the cost of hiring through an outside employment agency.

The salesperson in the OR during your procedure will be making suggestions to your surgeon on the use of their company's surgical instruments. Would you prefer a surgical salesperson with many years of surgical experience? Or a new-hire copier salesperson who had two weeks of product sales training and was then sent into the field to direct your surgeon on how to use an instrument that will affect your surgical outcome? The answer is quite obvious. Yet the standard business prototype for some surgical companies is to hire salespeople with no prior surgical or medical experience. In essence, they are potentially jeopardizing your safety.

When surgical companies look for new salespeople, some require that the new hire have several years' prior experience in surgical sales. This helps ensure that new employees have a solid OR background. Experienced salespeople know about proper OR technique. Nothing can replace experience and knowledge. That is vitally important in the OR. The new employees will be sent to the company training school to be trained on new instruments, equipment, and technology. However, it is a shorter learning curve for the experienced salespeople. They already know proper OR protocol.

Surgical companies have insurance liability policies on their salespeople and instruments. But does that really help a patient after surgical mishaps? Would the surgeon have more trust and feel more comfortable working with a salesperson who has several years of experience? Is there any justification for a company knowingly abiding by this type of policy?

In order to secure patient safety, I believe that there need to be standardized courses, testing, and appropriate certification for salespeople to enter the OR. Along with certification, there should be mandatory hours of continuing education training to maintain certification. Obviously, this certification should be a permanent record of achievement and be transferable. It would be a tremendous advantage and a credential on a resume for any salesperson seeking employment with a surgical corporation.

I have several final opinions about employment turnover in surgical corporations. Many surgical corporations believe in practicing management by intimidation and fear. These corporations think that employees will be more productive if they are threatened, harassed, and always scared about losing their jobs. I am at a point in my life where I cannot be intimidated with verbal threats of losing my job for lack of performance, losing business accounts, or declines in sales. It is not easy to intimidate an experienced, weathered salesperson. It is quite easy to do that to a young, inexperienced salesperson with a large mortgage and a young family.

From a financial standpoint, why retain an experienced salesperson who requires being paid a higher salary? It is easy to replace him with a younger representative that will command half the salary. And just as pertinent to this business culture and philosophy, I do not have blue eyes, long blond hair, and long legs.

The business culture, and, especially the health-care world of surgical manufacturers and suppliers, is obsessed with hiring young, attractive female employees. That is great if they are qualified. Regardless of sex, if a person is qualified, I think that he or she should not be discriminated against. I think that everyone should have the same opportunities. They should be paid the same wage for the same work effort, if the knowledge level and work experience are there.

Young, attractive female employees are eye candy to male purchasing agents, material managers, and surgeons. Men in a position of authority, regardless of their age, will always think that they have a chance with a young woman. They think that any woman views them as young, manly, and desirable. That is human nature, and it works more often than I chose to admit. And that thinking is a disservice to intelligent and dedicated working women, specifically. It is discrimination.

On the other hand, surgical companies are hiring young male employees to replace the older and experienced male sales veterans also. I believe in the same standard for them. If they are qualified, fine. They should be compensated for their talents and abilities on the same level. But why is there an obsession with youth over tempered experience, maturity, and the dedication to the work ethic that comes with age?

High employee turnover may also be associated with an employee's 401(K) plan.[1] Companies make yearly contributions to employees who establish a retirement plan. It has been said that the average length of employment with a company, regardless of whether the employee leaves or is terminated, is 2.4 years. As I understand, to be vested with a company and receive their full contributions to your plan, you have to be employed with them for at least five years. If the company terminates you before five years, or you leave, they may withdraw their contributions.[2] This is cruel, unethical, and calculated. It is designed to save millions of dollars in corporate contributions. And it happens to employees regularly. It is a practice that is endemic with corporate America.

I share these observations and offer these suggestions to help provide improved awareness and safety to patients. What I promote may provide a higher degree of insurance to hospitals, surgery centers, and surgeons. They would know that the surgical salespeople entering their facilities are not a threat to their patients. It would help reduce the potential that surgical corporations and their salespeople are providing misinformation on the use of technology that may lead to surgical mishaps.

I also encourage the surgical corporations of America to address their moral obligations and business ethics and how they relate to patient safety and surgical mishaps.

Chapter 2 Endnotes:

1. "Ultimate guide to retirement. How does a 401(k) plan work?," CNNMoney, accessed January 4, 2013, http://money.cnn.com/retirement/guide/401k_401kplans.moneymag/index.htm.
2. "Ultimate guide to retirement. How does vesting work?," CNNMoney, accessed January 4, 2013, http://money.cnn.com/retirement/guide/401k_401kplans.moneymag/index.htm?iid-EL.

Chapter 3
Understanding Hospitals

How Things Have Changed

The first hospital in the United States, Pennsylvania Hospital, was founded in 1751 by Dr. Thomas Bond and Benjamin Franklin. According to Bond and Franklin, the hospital was created "to care for the sick-poor and insane who were wandering the streets of Philadelphia."[1] At that time, this concept was quite a progressive idea. It was an idea based solely on doing compassionate mission work. It was received with enthusiasm and looked upon as a way to solve the health issues of all Americans.[2] It has been reported that Franklin later stated that he could not remember any political accomplishment that gave him as much pleasure as building that hospital.[3]

Since then, the number of hospitals has increased exponentially. Hospitals have increased the patient services provided, and there are varying types of hospitals. And, unfortunately, through the years the motives for establishing hospitals have progressed beyond simply doing compassionate mission work.

Today in the United States there are three types of hospitals. There are government hospitals, nonprofit hospitals, and for-profit hospitals.[4] The overwhelming majority of hospitals are nonprofit hospitals, with the number of government and for-profit hospitals being about the same.[5] Because of their different natures and requirements, each type of hospital is organized much differently, especially with regard to expenditures, receipts, budgets, and profitability. They may also differ in the patient services that they provide. Logically, the reason that a hospital will offer different, expanded, or limited services is based on their locale, size, and the type of administrative ownership.[6]

Although the three types of hospitals are different, there are a few ways in which they are all alike. First, all hospitals purchase medical devices from manufacturers and suppliers. They then mark up the cost of these devices to cover expenses and overhead. Depending on the type of hospital, that markup may be anywhere from a few percentage points to hundreds of times the original cost of the product.[7] Government hospitals usually have the least amount of markup. Nonprofit and for-profit hospitals have the higher markups.

Secondly, according to federal law, all hospitals must provide stabilizing care to anyone who walks into the facility.[8] Once a patient is stable, though, what happens to you next depends on the type of hospital that is treating you. Government hospitals will allow you to stay. With many patients, they do not charge for services. They absorb the patient health-care costs through city, county, state, or federal monies. "For-profit hospitals have the right to release patients whom the hospital believes may not be able to pay for treatment once stabilizing care has been administered. For-profit hospitals can refuse to treat patients with non-life-threatening illnesses or injuries because of a perceived inability to pay for treatment. This is not the case with nonprofit hospitals, which must treat all patients regardless of health insurance or financial status."[9]

Government Hospitals

Government and public hospitals may be city, county, state, or federally owned and operated. The money that is used to keep these facilities running and operational comes from city, county, state, or federal taxes. Regardless of how they are funded, they provide the same low-cost or cost-free services to all of their patients. With one exception, the VA hospitals only provide patient services to active and retired members of the military. However, direct family members may also qualify under a family plan that has reduced rates and provides for all medical and dental services.[10]

Government hospitals do their purchasing through one or more of the available purchasing programs. Those include GSA, FSS, DOD, VA, and some city, county, or state bidding programs. They are designed to help the member hospitals receive lower pricing through volume purchasing. Most of these purchasing agreements have specific requirements for their members and the medical suppliers. First, the medical supplier must be an approved government supplier. They must be on contract. The requirements include that the medical-supplier price offered to the government hospital is lower than that offered to private industry. The government gets the best price. Also, government pricing agreements state that hospitals must purchase American-made products over foreign-made products when possible.[11]

However, as the saying goes, some rules are made to be broken. I remember pricing situations where a medical supplier was charging a government hospital twice the price that was being charged to a nonprofit hospital. And, likewise, I remember countless situations where government hospitals did not follow the rules about buying American-made products on contract.

Several years ago, I was asked by the OR purchasing agent at one of my government hospitals to provide a proposal for a piece of OR equipment. A surgeon wanted this particular type of technology to be used in specific situations. The PA said that they were considering two of my competitors also. He told me the companies involved, and I realized that one of the competitors was a German manufacturer. When I mentioned this to him, he said that the hospital would make every attempt to purchase from one of the American manufacturers.

An evaluation period was scheduled for the surgeon to use each company's product to see which one he thought was superior. He also was interested in which company offered the best pricing. After the evaluation period, the surgeon said that all three companies' equipment was acceptable. He said that pricing would be crucial and the determining factor.

When I discovered who was awarded the bid, I was stunned. The German company won the business. The German equipment was priced at $38,000. My equipment was the lowest-priced product at $20,000. Purchasing my equipment would have saved the government $18,000. I sought out both the PA and the surgeon to discuss the reasons for the award being given to the German company. The PA would not give me a direct answer. He gave me several nonsensical excuses. I could see that he was embarrassed. The surgeon refused to meet with me. So much for the government buying the lowest-priced products and products made in America.

All government hospitals receive funding from one or more forms of government. The majority of patients seen in government or public hospitals are poor or impoverished people. The patients who are treated do not have to pay for their services if they cannot afford them. It is paid for by the government. If the patients qualify for Medicare or Medicaid, all, or a portion, of the treatment may be billed to Medicare or Medicaid.[12]

This type of payment or reimbursement system does not even come close to keeping government hospitals from losing money. The cost of health care has risen faster than the amount of reimbursement. And the rate of reimbursements further affects costs.

"As more advanced specialty treatments and procedures are performed, the cost of these procedures increases dramatically. There are medical advances, along with a longer life expectancy, an aging population and more people on government assistance and welfare. There are also an increasing number of retirees who do not pay into the system at a regular wage earners rate. They are using the services at a greater rate."[13] Plus, there is a cost associated with compliance to government regulations. As the number of regulations increase, the costs associated with regulations increase. One study stated that over 30 percent of every dollar spent in health care was spent on compliance to patient privacy regulations.[14] All of these factors have been squeezing the government system and adding to the drastic increase in health-care costs for years.

Government and public hospitals are underbudgeted and in financial difficulty. You would think that the fiscal mentality of management and administration would change to befit the situation. However, that is not the case. Every year, each department in the government hospitals is required to submit budget requests to the hospital administration for approval. Budgets are reviewed, approved, and then adjusted on a quarterly basis, in most facilities. Once budget money is approved and granted, every hospital department acquires a spend-it-or-lose-it mind-set. This means that if they do not spend the money that is available, their budgets may be reduced the next fiscal year. This has been an ongoing and ever-increasing problem, especially with the Veterans Administration hospitals.

I have been involved in buying situations in VA hospitals where money was spent on new equipment because the surgeon "just had to have the latest technology." The surgeon threatened to do more cases at other hospitals if the equipment was not purchased. The money was budgeted and approved for purchase on an emergency basis. The equipment was purchased, delivered, paid for, in-serviced, and then never used. Why? The surgeon moved to work at another facility. So the hospital was stuck with technology that other surgeons might not care to implement. This is a typical example of government fiscal irresponsibility at its worst.

There is another reason that government hospitals are having financial difficulties. It is the entire public union employment structure and work scale of government employees. Government employees are paid at an average rate that is much higher than that of private industry. It was recently reported that government employees earn an average of $30,000 per year more than workers in private industry. Once a government employee is hired and makes it past a work grace period, it is virtually impossible to have him or her terminated, for any cause. The more years that these employees work, the higher their GS grade becomes. Along with the grade-scale increase comes a mandatory pay-scale increase.

It has been reported that under several older government or public union retirement plans, employees did not have to contribute to their retirement or health-care programs. Those contributions were made by the taxpayer. Further, retiring with thirty years of service qualified them to receive 60 percent of their yearly salary. After forty-two years of service, their retirement was equal to about 80 percent of their yearly salary.

Based on a new program, the federal retirement scale rate is usually figured by taking the three highest salary years, multiply that by years of service and then multiply that by 1 percent.[15] After working over thirty years, many federal government retirees have a retirement pay that is much greater than private industry retirees.

Many federal workers' retirement pay is well into six figures. It makes no difference what their education level or job skill level is. And all of this is paid for by our taxes!

I remember hearing a recent news story. It reported that a public union employee received a yearly salary of over $150,000. He had a benefit package that included health care, dental, and retirement. And reportedly he contributed little or no portion of his salary to his health-care or retirement program. I believe that everyone has a right to earn as much money as possible. I have nothing against private union employees. They pay for their health and retirement programs. Why should public union employees receive special treatment? Why do members of public unions contribute nothing to retirement or health care? Why should the American taxpayer be responsible for this? This is the type of insanity that exists in government. And there are still people who ask why the United States is going broke.

The reality is that government and public hospitals are closing due to mismanagement, rising costs, and insufficient funds. A large part of the problem with insufficient funds is related directly to the increased burden of uninsured patients.[16] When the doors of the last government hospital close, where will the indigent, poor, and our veterans receive treatment? And what will be the service-cost increase and real tax increase for each working citizen to provide for that care?

Nonprofit Hospitals

Nonprofit hospitals account for the largest number of hospitals in the United States.[17] Many of them are associated with a religious institution, association, or order.[18] They usually have excellent reputations and are very well respected and received in their communities. Because they tend to be larger institutions, they provide a substantial number of excellent-paying jobs. And as a result of this, they have a powerful and impactful voice in the community.

Nonprofit hospitals are more likely to provide a wider range of services than government or public hospitals. In this manner, they are similar to for-profit hospitals. The larger the hospital, the wider the range of services provided.

Nonprofit hospitals operate under legal rules that are different than government or for-profit hospitals. They have a tax-exempt status and do not have to pay income, real estate, or sales taxes.[19] This is a huge benefit. Tax exemption provides the nonprofit hospital with more cash flow to expand the types of services provided, improve and update their facilities structures, and purchase equipment with the latest advancements in medical technology.[20]

If the nonprofit hospital is associated with a religious order, there is definitely a "mission" statement to which that hospital subscribes and follows. Those statements often profess that they exist to treat and heal the sick, that they save lives, that they will never turn anyone away, and that they will not charge for services if people cannot afford them. While this may be true, it is not the entire reason for their existence.

Anyone who thinks that nonprofit hospitals do not make money is not living in reality. Many are established on a corporate tax basis to not show a profit. However, nonprofit hospitals make tens or hundreds of millions of dollars a year. Much of that money is used for expansion and improvements. But much of it goes to administrators and board members that run the organization in the form of salaries, bonuses, and options. Some administrators and board members make millions of dollars a year in the name of healing and helping humanity.

The idea and purpose of health care started out to be a humanitarian effort to help mankind. It appears that the goal and direction has taken a backseat to the egotistical providers that have a thirst for power and money. Is this where the vision of Franklin has been taken?

I am saddened to say that it is. While for years the business world was filled with the personal corruption of greed, the health-care industry remained pristine and fully dedicated to healing. But, as with all ideals, reality injected its ugly head and tainted man's attempt at an honorable cause.

Nonprofit hospital national or regional associations often have dozens of members. These associations create GPOs or Group Purchasing Organizations.[21] They use their size to contract with medical manufacturers and suppliers to purchase products at reduced pricing. These contracts offer firm pricing for several years and may be a sole-source-provider agreement. If the agreements are sole source, the member hospitals must only use the products from that company. They have no flexibility in purchasing off contract. Sometimes, this helps the association to receive lower pricing. But it does not allow the individual hospital to make purchasing decisions.

Sometimes this type of restrictive and sole-source purchasing may actually drive up the cost of health care. I was working with several hospitals that belonged to one of the larger GPOs in the United States. Several surgeons specifically asked for surgical instruments from my company.

My products were not on their national agreement.

However, They were 15 to 20 percent lower than what they were paying for my competitor that was on contract. The hospitals talked to their local association contract manager to ask permission to purchase from me. They were told by their contract manager that they could not use my products. The surgeons were understandably frustrated and bewildered.

Later, I received a phone call from the contract manager of the association. She scheduled an appointment to meet with me. At that meeting, she was furious that I "had gone behind her back" to sell to her hospitals when I was not on contract. I explained that several surgeons had specifically requested to have my instruments and there would be a cost savings for her association of over $250,000 a year. She said that she did not care what the surgeons wanted. The doctors worked for her association, and they were not going to tell her what to purchase.

This is just one example of how the hospital side of the health-care system in the United States misses an opportunity to save money. How many times a day do these acts of stupidity (or as I refer to them, "acts of mental masturbation") occur? Is this an example of cronyism and graft? How much does this type of mismanagement or cronyism increase the cost of health care and jeopardize financial stability?

For-Profit Hospitals

For-profit hospitals are just what they say they are.

They are for profit. They are corporations that are in the health-care business, and they are run like any other free-market American company. They have an obligation to their investors and shareholders to turn a profit.[22] And that is their number-one concern. They sell shares of stock to investors and pay dividends on the earnings from those stocks.

The administrators and board of directors for these for-profit hospitals and corporations make millions of dollars. Unlike their counterparts in nonprofit hospitals, they not only admit it, they are proud of it. There is a certain amount of honesty that I appreciate in that.

The number of for-profit hospitals is growing in the United States. Many nonprofit hospitals are being purchased by for-profit hospital corporations.[23] The hospital corporations know the downfall of nonprofit hospitals. When nonprofit hospitals start to collapse from mismanagement of funds, the hospital corporation is ready to step in and buy. And they turn those hospitals into better money-making facilities.

Hospital corporations are better money managers and always stay within their budget allowances. Their facilities are usually located in more prominent neighborhoods where everyone has medical insurance. So even if the services that they provide are more costly, their patients can afford to pay.[24] These corporations are also shrewd at spending. They know that they will attract the better surgeons, who will have the opportunity to use the best in technology and make more money in the process. Hospital corporations are willing to pay top salaries for the better doctors.

Hospital corporations, like government and nonprofit hospitals, use their size to negotiate purchasing contracts with medical manufacturers and suppliers. The contracts that they agree to are usually single-source provider. They are multiyear in nature, usually for three to five years. And they will guarantee to the manufacturer that their corporation will use at least 90 percent of that manufacturer's product in all of their hospitals. This type of incentive to the manufacturer affords the hospital corporation the ability to achieve the lowest cost on products.

However, there is another suggested aspect, a negative aspect, to products that are purchased by some for-profit hospital corporations. It has been reported that some of these corporations purchase the cheapest-quality products available. These are products that may meet the minimum standards but could have questionable safety issues if used in procedural areas.

I remember working with the operating room PA in one of my for-profit hospitals. The facility was purchasing one of my products, and he wanted to know if I could sell it to them at a lower price. I told him that the price was a contract price and could not be changed. He said that he would try to find a less expensive product.

After receiving price quotes from other suppliers, he told me that the hospital OR was switching to a product that was made in China. I was familiar with that particular product. That product did have FDA[25] approval. However, I knew that it reportedly had caused some fires in the OR because of a lack of proper insulation. When I informed the PA of this, he said, "That's okay. We will be saving so much money that I don't care. We will worry about that if and when it happens." I could not believe what I was hearing. He was saying that saving the hospital corporation money was more important than the safety of the patients in their OR.

University and Teaching Hospitals

Teaching hospitals and university hospitals are extremely complex organizations. There are layers of nurses, interns, residents, instructors, associate professors, professors, fellows, master of science degree holders, PhDs, chairmen, and MDs. The hospital may or may not be associated with a university. If it is associated with a university, it will be called a university hospital.[26] These are hospitals that perform operations, and their main purpose is to be a training facility for doctors, medical students, and nurses.

These institutions have large endowment funds and are awarded grant money from the government and private industry. It has been reported that one of the larger medical schools in the United States has an endowment fund worth over $32 billion. With this amount of money, teaching hospitals are able to purchase medical and surgical technology that is the finest in the world. And with that money there is investment in research and the ability to pioneer new surgical techniques. They are also able to pay their staff members the highest salaries.

Not all teaching hospitals have endowment funds of this size. However, most are in the range of hundreds of millions of dollars. Knowing this, why do these institutions receive government grants, research funds, corporate donations, and tax exemptions? I think that it is obscene to do so. It is no different than giving billionaires that own professional sports teams tax abatements to build and operate their stadia. I have passionate feelings about that, as well.

Many medical manufacturers and private corporations make large contributions to the endowment funds of these hospitals on a yearly basis. And the corporations that make contributions expect something in return. They expect the hospital to use the surgical products that they manufacture and sell. It is a perfect quid pro quo situation.

I remember working in the animal lab at a prestigious university hospital. The animal lab is where surgeons operate on animals to hone their skills, attempt new procedures, and evaluate new technology and instruments before they use them on humans. There were three surgeons using my company's equipment. I was there to answer any questions that they might have about the products' capabilities. I was also interested in showing them new instrumentation that I had available. I wanted to increase my sales.

As I went into my sales pitch, one of the surgeons

quickly stopped me. He said, "Curt, we currently use your competitor, who donates $3 million a year to our school of medicine. What can your company do for us?" I told him that I understood, and I thanked him for letting me know.

I never approached that surgeon again. I could not compete with a company that was donating millions every year to a university hospital to buy its business support. My company could not afford to do business that way. And, once more, the instruments that I wanted him to consider were of superior quality and lower in price.

Teaching hospitals are necessary in the development and training of surgeons. However, they have been under close scrutiny and criticism. Often, the "surgeon" operating on you is a trainee that is working under the supervision of a resident or attending surgeon. There has been suggestion that this makes teaching hospitals less safe and that there is a greater risk for mistakes to occur due to the surgeon trainee's lack of experience.[27] Whether this is true will always be up for discussion and debate.

I will say that from my own personal experience, having observed hundreds of surgeries in teaching hospitals, if you choose to have surgery in a teaching hospital, make sure that the residents only observe. Request that the procedure be done "skin to skin" by the attending physician. This will ensure that the resident will learn from observing. It may also reduce the potential that a mistake will be made at the expense of your health and well-being.

Surgery Centers and Outpatient Surgery Centers

Surgery centers are the fastest-growing type of surgical procedural center in the United States. They may be a freestanding facility located in a mall or shopping center area. Or they may be an outpatient surgery center located on the grounds of a hospital. They may be hospital owned, doctor owned, or corporately owned. They may be for-profit or nonprofit. And, like hospitals, the type of ownership may make a difference in the cost of the procedure and the level and type of patient care given.

What is the definition and purpose of a surgery center? A surgery center is "designed for procedures that can be done outside of a hospital, usually without an overnight stay. Most specialize in just a few specific, or even just a single area of practice, such as eyes, hand, heart, joints, cosmetic surgery, etc. Their growth in popularity comes from the improved technology that allows these procedures to be done outside of the hospital, plus the more luxurious settings that these facilities often provide."[28]

It is estimated that approximately 65 percent of all surgical procedures are performed on an outpatient basis, both at hospitals and in surgery centers.[29] The number has been growing every year since the inception of the surgery center concept more than thirty years ago.

Whether to have surgery in the OR of a hospital, hospital outpatient surgery center, or surgery center is a serious decision and needs careful thought. There are positives and negatives to each.

There are several conveniences to surgery centers and outpatient surgery centers. They are easier to access than hospitals. You do not have to worry about the hassle of parking garages, as in large hospitals. They are smaller, cozier, and more comfortable. They are facilities that are not logistically confusing. They are not as intimidating as hospitals.

Quite often, the cost of having a surgical procedure performed in a surgery center or outpatient surgery center is appreciably less. One recent study compared the costs of various procedures done at a surgery center to those at a hospital. The study discovered that a surgical procedure performed at a surgery center cost 47 percent less than one performed at a full-service hospital.[30]

On the other hand, I have two major concerns regarding surgery centers and outpatient surgery centers. They are infection control and the potential need for emergency treatment.

In hospitals, there is a specific nurse (or team of nurses) with the title of infection control nurse. In many states, nurses must take courses and become certified and licensed to practice infection control.

The entire responsibility of this nurse or team is to promote infection control. They monitor all patient and nonpatient areas. They are regularly testing, sampling, and culture plating all hospital departments. They conduct regular in-services with all hospital staffs on the standards and universal precautions regarding infection control. Their expertise and work greatly reduces the risk of a patient acquiring a nosocomial infection, or, an infection that is a result of treatment in a medical facility. Infection control is a serious, costly, and monumental task.

Many surgery centers and outpatient surgery centers do not have the personnel or the resources to do infection control monitoring at the same level as hospitals. Often, the person in charge of infection control at a surgery center has other jobs too.[31] The turnaround times between surgeries are shorter.[32] There is less time to disinfect the OR between procedures. During recent years, there has been an alarming increase in postoperative infections found at surgery centers. Yet surgery centers need to be held to the same standards of infection control as hospitals.[33]

My second concern with having surgery at a surgery center or outpatient surgery center is regarding emergencies. With any surgical procedure there is the risk of needing emergency treatment. Surgery centers do not have the necessary equipment to handle all emergency situations. If emergency treatment is delivered at a surgery center, the patient may still need to be transferred to a hospital and placed in an intensive care or surgical intensive care unit.

If you have surgery performed at a hospital and require emergency treatment, you are already in the hospital. Hospitals have the most sophisticated emergency equipment available. Most intensive care and surgical intensive care units are located adjacent to the hospital OR suite. If you need to be transferred to a specialty unit, it only takes moments. The ability to save time in emergencies cannot be overemphasized. Time saved is a life saved.

There are differences in the types of hospitals and surgery centers available. You have options to consider. Make sure that you do your research into the hospital or surgery center that you may enter. It may make the difference in the level of patient care that you receive and in your surgical outcome.

Chapter 3 Endnotes:

1. "The Story of the Creation of the Nation's First Hospital," Penn Medicine, accessed December 9, 2012, http://www.uphs.upenn.edu/paharc/features/creation.html.
2. Ibid.
3. Ibid.
4. Jill Horowitz, "Making Profits and Providing Care: Comparing Nonprofit, For-Profit, and Government Hospitals," University of Michigan Law School, accessed December 5, 2012, http://content.healthaffairs.org/content/24/3/790.full.
5. Ibid.
6. Ibid.
7. Ames Alexander, Karen Garloch, and Joseph Neff, "Nonprofit Hospitals Thrive on Profits," *Charlotte Observer,* April 21, 2012, http://www.charlotteobserver.com/2012/04/21/318921/nonprofit-hospitals-thrive-on.html.
8. Jonathan Lister, "For-profit Vs. Nonprofit Hospitals," eHow, accessed December 5, 2012, http://www.ehow.com/info_7742145_forprofit-vs-nonprofit-hospitals.html.
9. Ibid.
10. "Health Benefits," United States Department of

Veterans Affairs, August 15, 2012, http://www.va.gov/healthbenefits/access/family_members.asp.

11. "GSA Schedules," US General Services Administration, August 29, 2012, http://www.gsa.gov/portal/content/197989; Angela Ogunjimi, "How to Achieve and Use a GSA Schedule," eHow, accessed December 5, 2012, http://www.ehow.com/how_5129474_achieve-use-gsa-schedule.html; Kit Tunstall, "Requirements for Department of Defense Contracts," eHow, accessed December 5, 2012, http://www.ehow.com/list_6833538-definitions-department-defense-contractor.html; "Prospective Contractors," Department of Veterans Affairs, December 27, 2011, http://www.va.gov/oal/business/fss/prospective.asp.27Dec.

12. "What Medicare Covers," Medicare.gov, accessed January 26, 2013, http://medicare.gov/what-medicare-covers/index.html; "Medicaid Program," Medicaid Program.net, accessed January 26, 2013, http://www.medicaidprogram.net.

13. "Publicly Funded Health Care," Wikipedia, December 26, 2012, http://en.wikipedia.org/wiki/Publicly_funded_healthcare.

14. "Addressing Regulatory Compliance in the Healthcare Industry," NetIQ, January 2006, http://download.netiq.com/CMS/WHITEPAPER/NetIQIndustryWP_HC.pdf.

15. Mark Cussen, "How to Calculate FERS Retirement," eHow, accessed December 6, 2012, http://www.

ehow.com/how_5180814_calculate-fers-retirement.html.

16. "Public Hospital," Wikipedia, November 14, 2012, http://en.wikipedia.org/wiki/Public_hospital.

17. "Non-Profit Hospital," Wikipedia, October 17, 2011, http://en.wikipedia.org/wiki/Non-profit_hospital.

18. Ibid.

19. Horowitz, "Making Profits and Providing Care: Comparing Nonprofit, For-Profit, and Government Hospitals."

20. Alexander, Garloch, and Neff, "Nonprofit Hospitals Thrive on Profits."

21. "Group Purchasing Organization," Wikipedia, January 6, 2013, http://en.wikipedia.org/wiki/Group_purchasing_organization.

22. "For-Profit Hospital," Wikipedia, November 20, 2012, http://en.wikipedia.org/wiki/For-profit_hospital.

23. Lister, "For-Profit Vs. Nonprofit Hospitals."

24. Horowitz, "Making Profits and Providing Care: Comparing Nonprofit, For-Profit, and Government Hospitals."

25. "Medical Devices," FDA, December 31, 2012, http://content.healthaffairs.org/content/24/3/790.full.

26. Jessica Ellis, "What Is a Teaching Hospital?," wiseGEEK, accessed January 11, 2013, http://www.wiseGEEK.com/what-is-a-teaching-hospital.htm.

27. Ellis, "What Is a Teaching Hospital?"

28. "Surgery Centers," Anthem Education, accessed January 11, 2013, http://www.careercollege.edu/Career-Opportunities/Surgery-Centers/.

29. Ibid.

30. Chris Harmen, "Surgery Center Versus Hospital—Which Is Preferred?," Ezine Articles, accessed January 11, 2013, http://ezinearticles.com/?Surgery-Center-Versus-Hospital---Which-is-Preferred?&id=397.

31. "Inspectors Cite Illinois Surgery Centers," Associated Press, August 8, 2011, http://www.stltoday.com/news/national/article_9d992d42-ade9-52e0-8933-61df7600b0ec.

32. Ibid.

33. Ibid.

Chapter 4
The Operating Room Suite

A Place I Call Home

The operating room suite is comprised of operating rooms. The number of ORs, as they are referred to, in the suite differs depending on the size of the hospital. That number is usually based on the number of beds or patient rooms. A one-hundred-bed hospital may only have two ORs while the average three-hundred-bed hospital could have ten ORs or more. It is not uncommon for the larger teaching or university hospitals to have over one thousand beds or patient rooms and have in excess of fifty ORs. In these facilities, there may be a separate floor or group of ORs that are dedicated to a specific service. This practice is especially true for services specializing in women's care, cancer treatment, open heart, and orthopedics.

In small hospitals, the types of surgical services provided are sometimes limited. The usual procedures performed are general; orthopedics; ear, nose, and throat; some urology; colonoscopies; and gynecological. Each OR may be used to perform all types of procedures.

In larger hospitals, the ORs are usually designated according to the different types of surgical services that are performed. Those services include a much greater array and offer much more specialized and higher technological care. Designating each OR for a specific service reduces the need to move equipment from room to room between cases. It also allows the OR supply shelves, in that room, to be stocked with related items for that service only.

As you enter the suite, in the main corridor, there is usually a surgery scheduling desk. And there are several department nurses at that desk to meet and observe all who enter. There is great concern about who is entering the suite for safety, infection control, and privacy issues.

Until several years ago, it was very easy for anyone to gain access and enter the OR. Now there are a series of steps taken for people other than patients and staff to gain entry. Those other people would include sales representatives that work for medical/surgical companies in procedural or patient-care areas.

Most hospitals subscribe to a credentialing service. For a yearly fee, that service will handle the necessary requirements, for the hospital, to ensure that all salespeople entering procedural or patient-care areas are registered and safe to enter. These credentialing services will also charge the medical companies a yearly fee for every sales representative to ensure that they meet all standards.

The credentialing process requires that representatives receive all and any disease inoculations. It also requires that salespeople take a drug test, have a background check, show proof of appropriate procedural training and certification, and have a letter from their company showing that they have corporate liability insurance and are bonded.

Once all requirements are verified, the credentialing service will register that representative. Each time that representatives want access to any procedural or patient-care area, they will go to a kiosk. At the kiosk, they enter their e-mail address and password. If they are up-to-date with their requirements, they will be issued a badge for a specific amount of time for that day. The badge is only good for that day, the amount of time specified on the badge, and the specified area.

The salesperson must wear that badge in plain view at all times while in the facility. Departmental and security personnel are told to look for these badges. If you do not display one, it is considered a violation of hospital policy. You will be stopped and sent to material management to be counseled. Two or three violations in one hospital could result in the sales representative being permanently barred from entering or working in that institution. The company for whom the representative works is also notified. This may result in the sales representative being terminated.

The hospital credentialing services provide a necessary

and vital program for all involved in health care. They help protect the hospital from unnecessary, unqualified, and potentially infectious people entering patient-care and procedural areas. They protect the patients from acquiring nosocomial infections and from unqualified personnel working with their doctors. And they help protect salespeople from potential disease, infection, and legal litigation.

Across from the surgery desk, there is usually a surgery schedule board that has the OR room numbers, the type of surgeries scheduled for each room that day, and which nurses and doctors are working in that room. The surgery board may also have other pertinent information to read related to health-care and OR specific topics.

As you move along the main OR corridor, you will notice a red line on the floor. This line is not to be crossed unless you are in OR scrub attire. You will find doors before this line that lead to the men's and women's locker rooms. These locker room areas are where the staff and visitors change into the surgical scrubs, shoe covers, and head covers that need to be worn, at all times, while in the OR suite. Once you change into OR attire, there is another exit door on the far side of the locker room. This door will take you to the other side of the red line and give you access to the individual ORs.

Besides the OR rooms, the suite contains a main storage room for equipment. This room stores all equipment when it is not is use. The equipment room is normally quite large. There is not only a vast variety of equipment. There are multiple numbers of each type. If a hospital has ten operating rooms, there may be ten units of each type of equipment being stored. Each piece of equipment is numbered by the hospital, inventoried in the computer, and inspected on a regular maintenance program. The regular maintenance program ensures the working integrity of each unit.

There will also be a main storeroom where sterile disposable supplies, sterile instruments, and instrument trays are stored. This area is also known as the central sterile supply in some institutions. This area may only be entered if you are wearing a surgical mask. These central sterile areas may contain sterilizers where instruments are processed. Most hospitals, though, have a separate area called sterile processing where instruments are cleaned, decontaminated, placed in trays, wrapped, labeled, dated, and then sterilized. If this sterile processing area is outside the OR, after sterilization, the instruments are returned to a central sterile supply area in the OR.

Contained in the OR suite, also, are a nurses' lounge and a surgeons' lounge. The nurses' lounge is usually available to all surgical sales representatives. It is a prime area to conduct in-services and demonstrations on instruments or equipment, to set up informational displays, or to relax between cases.

The surgeons' lounge is a different story. It is forbidden to salespeople unless they have an invitation from a surgeon. Even with an invitation, most surgeons do not appreciate or want salespeople in their lounge. Some hospitals will have a surgeons' dining area off of the surgeons' lounge. This allows the surgeons the privacy that they want and believe that they deserve. If the surgeons' lounge does not have a dining area, there will be one adjacent to the main dining area in the hospital. The rules are the same for that dining area. Only surgeons are allowed. And the sign on the door will tell you that.

The ORs are usually on either side of the main corridor and numbered or lettered. Usually, between two ORs on the same side of the corridor will be a scrub sink where the nurses and surgeons scrub their hands with an approved surgical scrub solution before they enter the room. Above these sinks you will also find surgical masks that are to be worn before scrubbing their hands and entering the OR. Often, there may be a substerile room between the two ORs. This room will have a small sterilizer to flash instruments, a blanket warmer, and other small OR equipment. This room will have an entrance to the OR and is the preferred way to gain access into the OR. Most hospital OR nursing staffs will not allow personnel to enter any OR room from the main corridor.

Inside each OR room will be a variety of medical equipment, depending on which type of service that room is delegated to perform. The standard equipment in every OR, regardless of the type of service, includes the OR table, OR lights, X-ray equipment, and screens, anesthesia equipment, cautery equipment, TV video towers, power cords, supply shelves, waste containers, intercom service, and a computer kiosk. There may be other smaller procedural devices.

Two other patient-care areas are usually found within the OR suite. They are preoperative holding and postoperative holding.

Preoperative holding is where the patient is taken before his or her surgical procedure. It is an area where the final preparations are made before the patient enters a specific operating room. A nurse will escort the patient to a small, curtained changing area or private room. The patient will change from street clothes into a hospital gown. The patient will then be asked a myriad of questions including name; health history; all prescription drugs, nonprescription drugs, or herbal supplements being taken; what procedure is to be done; and the name of the doctor. It will be necessary to fill out, complete, and sign all paperwork and surgical consent forms.

At this time, an IV line will be placed in a vein in his or her arm or hand. This IV will be used during their surgery to administer anesthesia and any other medications, or fluids, if necessary. Someone from the anesthesia department, a nurse or a doctor, will visit to ask if he or she has any questions about being put to sleep during the procedure. The medical professional will also answer any questions about the type of anesthesia that will be administered. The surgical staff knows how important it is for the patient to be relaxed before the procedure. Often, the nurse anesthetist or the anesthesiologist will administer a preoperative sedative through the IV line. The preop sedative helps the patient relax.

People have different reactions to medications. The reaction to preop sedatives is no different. I have seen and heard strange and laughable behavior from patients after their sedatives. I have heard people start singing like birds. I have heard people start telling stories about their relatives, friends, girlfriends or boyfriends, and mistresses. I even heard a convict from one of the prisons start talking about the people that he had shot some years before. I have seen people try to get off of the transport stretcher and want to go home. You never know what that preop sedative will make a person do or say.

Finally, the last person to visit the patient in preop will be his or her surgeon. The surgeon will verify what surgery the patient is having and will answer any questions that the patient has about his or her surgery. The final thing that the surgeon will do is mark the surgical site, usually with his/her initials.

When the patient is ready for surgery, and the surgical room is available, the patient will be taken to the room on a transport stretcher. Once inside the OR itself, the OR team will begin their assigned duties to prepare the patient and perform the procedure under the guidance of the attending surgeon. Team members are well trained in their fields of expertise and know how to work together in harmony. They will work the procedure together from start to finish.

The OR team is led by the attending surgeon. The

attending surgeon makes all decisions on everything that transpires during that procedure. The surgeon has total responsibility and is fully liable. The rest of the OR team usually consists of the circulating room nurse, the scrub tech or techs (some types of procedures require more than one scrub tech), the nurse anesthetist or anesthesiologist, sometimes an assisting surgeon or resident, and a surgeon's assistant. There also may be several surgical salespeople in the room.

The surgical salesperson is in the OR to answer any questions that the surgeon may have about the application of his or her instrument or equipment. They *do not* have any hands-on treatment with a patient. Only medically trained and certified personnel at the OR table, under the surgeon's watchful supervision and instruction, will apply hands to a patient. The stories that have circulated about salespeople actually doing surgery are not true. They are ridiculous!

The postoperative holding area is where surgical patients are taken immediately after their surgery is completed. During his or her time in this area, as in the OR during surgery, the patient is constantly monitored. The amount of time spent in recovery depends on how quickly the patient recovers from the effects of anesthesia, the stability of his or her vital signs, and his or her bodily functions.

At the time of release from recovery, an in-house patient will be assigned to a room. An outpatient will be discharged to return home. The discharged patient will only be released to a relative or friend after signing release forms.

All ORs are terminally disinfected by the OR housekeeping staff on a regular basis. The OR housekeeping staff is trained for this duty and is dedicated to only clean and disinfect the OR. It is a job of vital importance. This process includes floors, walls, and every piece of equipment in the room. That schedule includes disinfection between procedures and a final terminal disinfection at the end of the day. The purpose is to prevent surgical patients from acquiring nosocomial or postoperative infections. It also provides a clean, healthy work environment for the hospital staff.

The OR suite is the engine that drives the hospital. It is the single greatest revenue-producing department in the hospital. Because of this, the OR budget in most hospitals is also very large. The hospital administrators know that a modern and efficient operating room is a great public relations tool to attract doctors and patients. I have seen operating room facilities in small towns that are as well equipped and staffed as any of the well-known facilities in large metropolitan areas. People in outstate areas do not have to leave their hometowns to receive quality health care.

I believe that there is a difference between the OR in the small-town hospital and the OR in a large metropolitan-area hospital. It has to do with the administration of patient care. I have always had a closer identity with the ORs in small-town community hospitals. The nurses and doctors seem to have a more caring attitude toward their patients. In small towns, everyone knows each other. The patient is a relative, a friend, or a friend of a relative. As a result, there is more of a natural bond between caregiver and patient. The surgeons are there because they care more about their patients than making the money available to them in large hospitals. Not that the care given in large hospitals is inadequate, but there is an emotional disconnect between patient and caregiver in the larger facilities. That is true of nurses and surgeons alike.

I find that small-town hospital OR staffs are friendlier toward surgical salespeople. The nurses are genuinely interested to see new technology and instrumentation, and they conduct regular in-services for continuing education credits. The surgeons are friendlier and more approachable. They will give you time to discuss new medical technology without having to buy lunch. They do not seem to have the egos. In many larger hospitals, you have a sense that neither the OR nurses nor the surgeons want you there.

Chapter 5
OR Nurses and Surgical Technicians

The True Caregivers

I have the utmost respect and highest regard for the nurses and surgical technicians that work in the OR. They are the most professional, hardworking, and caring group with whom I have ever been associated. The nurses and surgical technicians have different titles, job duties, and responsibilities. But they work together as a team to provide patient care before, during, and after a surgical procedure. They are the champions of the OR.

The titles of the nurses in the OR vary from hospital to hospital. The nurse who runs the OR is called the director of surgery, nurse manager, or OR supervisor. She is the administrative coordinator for nurses, techs, and surgeons. In larger hospitals, there may also be a head nurse who is in charge of each particular service, (i.e., head nurse of orthopedics). The head nurse is responsible for making sure that supplies for that service are ordered and maintained. They are also responsible for all circulating nurses and scrub technicians that work in that service. The head nurse takes care of problems and issues related to her service. They are hands-on managers.

The circulating nurse is a registered nurse and is the nurse who supervises the entire OR during surgery. She is not dressed with a sterile gown and gloves. So she is the coordinator between nonsterile and sterile fields. Before surgery, the circulator checks the working condition of all equipment that will be used and gathers the necessary packaged supplies for the procedure. She will work in unison with the sterile scrub tech to open packages and trays for placement in the sterile fields.

When the patient is brought into the OR on a stretcher, it is the circulating nurse who takes charge and administers to the needs of the patient. She will do a nursing assessment, ensure the patient identity, and qualify all pertinent and necessary information about the patient that is needed before surgery.

The circulator is responsible for all patient charge entries into the computer. Those entries include all standard charge items and any add-on products that are later used. She is also responsible for completing any and all patient paperwork and forms. If there is any verbal or written communication from parties outside the OR, the circulator will relay messages to the team at the OR table.

The circulator ensures that the sterile surgical team at the OR table has the necessary sterile surgical supplies. The circulator is able to take sterile, packaged items from the nonsterile areas of the OR, open them, and hand them to the scrub nurse for placement in sterile surgical areas. This is done without comprising the sterile integrity of the instrument, supply, or the field itself. All supplies and instruments that enter the sterile field are counted by the circulator, and a record is kept. A final count of all instruments and supplies is made twice during the procedure between the circulator and the scrub.

It is the circulator's responsibility to constantly watch for any breaks of integrity in the sterile fields that are established in the OR. Those sterile areas are the surface of the OR table, any surface that has open sterile instruments or supplies, and the OR team standing at the OR table. If there is any compromise in sterility observed by the circulator, she will take measures to reestablish the sterile field.

When the surgical procedure is completed, it is the circulating nurse who transports the patient to the postoperative recovery area. She will return to the OR and start getting ready for the next procedure after the OR is disinfected.

Before the procedure, the scrub technician, or scrub, is responsible for collecting and opening all instrument trays. Once trays are opened, she will leave the room and scrub her hands at the OR sink. She will return to the room and put on a sterile gown and sterile gloves. Once this step is completed, she can only touch sterile items. Her coordinator for introducing packaged sterile items for placement into the sterile field is the circulator.

Now, the scrub will take instruments out of the sterile trays and arrange them for use during the procedure. She will count all instruments, sponges, blades, needles, sutures, and ancillary products.

She will keep a count of these items and relay that count to the circulating nurse. She will discuss these counts with the circulator twice before the procedure has ended. All instruments and supplies used must be accounted for when the procedure is finished and before the patient leaves the room.

The scrub works in tandem with the circulating nurse from the sterile field. The scrub is also responsible for the handling and transferring of all sterile supplies that are used by the surgeon during the procedure. She will place instruments in and out of the field as they are requested by the surgeon. The scrub is responsible for monitoring the integrity of the sterile field at the OR table. If she notices any break in sterile integrity, it is her responsibility to remove the compromised items and reestablish the sterile field. If the surgeon needs an item that is not in the field or in the trays, the scrub will request that the circulator retrieve that supply and transfer it to her.

During the procedure, the scrub will assist the surgeon in holding instruments and retractors, positioning scopes, suctioning fluids, and wiping off instruments after each use. She is an extra set of hands, eyes, and ears for the surgeon.

When the procedure is finished and the patient has left the room, the scrub transports the used instrument trays to the central sterile decontamination room for reprocessing. She will return to the OR and wait to set up for the next procedure.

Besides their regular duties, the breadth of issues that the OR nursing staff tolerates on a daily basis is inconceivable. They must deal with tantrums, egos, complaining, arguments, lecturing, yelling, screaming, cursing, laughing, sexual harassment, and outright meanness. Walk into any OR during surgery, and you will hear a myriad of verbal trash and crap that will make you cringe. It is usually directed at one or more of the nurses or scrubs. And all of it is coming from the surgeons doing the procedure.

The depth and extent of the abuse from the surgeon is directly related to his disposition that day. There are times when the atmosphere in the OR is great and everyone is in a good mood. Music is playing, and conversation is light and amusing. The procedure is going well. Unfortunately, those times are infrequent. I find most surgeons to be highly qualified in their medical skills and knowledge. They rate embarrassingly low on their people skills.

I marvel at OR nurses and scrubs. They perform a critical job with professionalism and dedication. Their work requires a higher level of responsibility. Often, they perform under extreme and stressful circumstances. They have an amazing understanding and knowledge of how to operate electrical equipment, machinery, drills, cameras, scopes, and every tool that is imaginable. Much of what they know is learned in the classroom. They spend a lot of time in training programs, lectures, and in-services earning contact credits to maintain their licenses and certifications.

OR nurses and scrubs are mentally tough and are not easily shaken. It is a necessity that they have this temperament to handle the high level of stress and responsibility of the OR. They are always upbeat and positive. They won't shy away from any surgical responsibility or wilt under any pressure. They are professionals who know their roles and how to work as a team. But, most importantly, they are sensitive and caring and have hearts of gold.

They are the true caregivers.

Chapter 6
Surgeons

They Are Who They Are

Becoming a surgeon is not easy. It is a long and difficult educational process. It takes a great amount of time, money, and dedication. Much personal sacrifice is needed to reach that pinnacle of success.

Education Portal says, "The educational requirements are 4 years of undergraduate school at a university or college graduating with a B.S. or B.A. Entrance exams must be taken for acceptance into medical school. Medical school is also 4 year educational programming, after which, you are a physician. However, you need to complete a residency program before you may practice surgery on your own. The residency program will take 3–7 years, depending on the specialty that is pursued. After residency, you are now a surgeon that has the ability to operate on your own. However, if you want to become highly specialized in your field, you may want to do a fellowship. Fellowship programs take 1–3 years, again, depending on your field of study."[1]

There is a lot of prestige associated with being a surgeon. Surgeons complete a grueling and respected education schedule. They spend a lot of money to accomplish their goal and attain their degrees. They are gifted and skilled at their profession. They make a lot of money (which I believe most of them earn honestly). And, because of their supposed stature, they have business and social opportunities available to them that most people will never have.

Ideal surgeons are ones who follow the path that they pledge to walk. They take an oath to do no harm or injustice to anyone. They pledge to be just and true in their life and profession. These are honorable intentions for an honorable cause. However, the purity and the ideal of the profession is becoming lost. It has taken a seat behind the front of fame and fortune. The content of the oath has changed many times during the last hundred years to accommodate attitudes in societal issues and politics. Its strict resolve has been adapted to allow for the convenience of a clear conscience. Accordingly, it is my understanding that the majority of surgeons do not even take the oath upon graduation from medical school. Do they not want to pledge to a philosophy or way of life in which they do not believe?

There is a certain aura and mystique about surgeons. I think that it is enhanced because they are aloof and difficult to know. They only associate with other doctors and attempt to keep their personal lives very private. Try to engage a surgeon in conversation if you see him walking down the hallway in an operating room setting. He will usually try to ignore you and just keep walking. Yet people seem to place them on pedestals and hold them in such curiously high esteem. They are revered.

I am always amused at how they are believed to be completely honorable and above reproach. But why is that? Is it because they have the title of surgeon? They are no better or worse than any of us. In fact, I believe that many grew up with antisocial personalities. They were the kids who were the nerds in elementary and secondary school. They were the last ones picked on the sports teams. They made excellent grades and possessed genius capabilities but never quite fit in with the others. They had few friends. They were sheepish and shy.

I think that their whole persona changed with maturity and medical school. They found their calling in life. Becoming a surgeon made them realize the power and authority that they possess. It gave them confidence and poise. The change has also given them narcissistic personalities. They carry themselves in ways that suggest that they are above others. They are arrogant, pompous, and unapproachable.

The daily surgery schedule in the OR is well planned and allows for few delays or last-minute changes. If changes or delays occur, nurses and anesthesia may have to stay late and work overtime. Overtime pay in the OR costs hospitals large sums of money. There is also a charge associated with using the OR. The charge per minute for OR time varies from $22 to $133 per minute, depending on the type and magnitude of the procedure.[2] Surgeons are notorious for being late to the OR. They have no regard for when their surgeries are scheduled to start. It is not uncommon for a surgeon to be thirty minutes late to the hospital for the start of his procedure. A thirty-minute delay could cost the OR an extra $660–$3,990 in profits per procedure.

This lackadaisical attitude by surgeons over being late happens every day. It drives the OR nurse management crazy. And it is not just one surgeon who is constantly late. Many make it their habit. Very seldom will they call the OR scheduler to say that they are going to be late. And do not ask why they were late or did not call. They will verbally undress you.

During a surgical procedure, the surgeon is in charge. And he or she should be. The surgeon is the person with full liability. I usually do not question a surgeon's skills or medical proficiency. Most are excellent clinicians. Although, I have seen surgeons perform procedures as if they had never worked a case before. They make all the decisions without being questioned. The surgeon is always right. To question a surgeon is to be thrown out of the operating room. In all of the surgeries that I have witnessed, I have only heard a few admissions of guilt or wrongdoing on their part.

Surgeons have poor communication skills. The manner in which they talk to the OR staff and product salespeople during a surgical procedure can be shameful. They talk with a level of disdain. They cannot accept when things do not go their way. When nurses do not hand them an instrument in a particular manner or hold a retractor to their liking, you will hear the beast within emerge. The personal insults and demeaning tone of voice used to correct and scold will belittle the most experienced OR nurse.

For the surgical salesperson, your instrument and your instructions on how to use it must be perfect. Surgeons have very quick tempers if they cannot adapt quickly to an instrument or technique. If they do not, it means a quick exit for both of you.

Surgeons receive special treatment in the hospital, in the operating room, in their office, and in public life. They have their own special lounges, dining areas, and hospital parking spaces. All of their meals are paid for by the hospital, some medical/surgical company, or pharmaceutical supplier. They belong to the finest country clubs. They have money for exclusive travel, buy the nicest homes and automobiles, have season tickets to sporting events, and send their children to the best schools. Yet they seem to be an unhappy group of people. You very seldom see them smile or laugh.

I have categorized surgeons into five basic types of personalities. They are the academician, the complainer, the new-toy surgeon, the leave-me-alone surgeon, and the humanitarian. There are others, but these make up the majority.

The Academician

Academicians are surgeons who love to teach, to pontificate, and to hear themselves talk. They want everyone to know how smart they are. They have profound titles and enough letters after their names to fill an alphabet. They are not only found in academia; they are in every hospital. They love to travel and lecture at seminars and conferences. And, of course, they do not lecture for free. They accept rather large stipends for their services so that you may learn of their incredible insight and brilliance. I believe that they care more about their reputations and positions in the surgical society than they do about delivering patient care.

They also feel the need to lecture and correct everyone working in the OR during their procedures. They are never at a loss for words and never lecture without their self-indulgent egos present.

I remember working a particular case with an academician. He talked and lectured the entire time that he was operating. When the procedure was over, he finished closing the incision with suture and asked the scrub nurse to cut some adhesive strips into lengths of one and a half inches. He would place them across the incision before the bandage was placed over the wound. When she gave him the adhesive strips, he quickly called for a ruler. He did not think that the strips were the right length. He measured the strips and found that they were one-eighth inch too long. He lectured her for ten minutes about not listening to him and how important it is to follow his explicit instructions.

I have specific instructions for those considering surgery. Stay away from this egomaniac. At one time, he probably was a skilled surgeon who really cared for his patients. Unfortunately, he has progressed on to feeding his idea of self-worth.

The Complainer

The complainer drives you crazy. The moment that he walks through the door of the OR it begins. As he is gowning and gloving he is looking at everything with a disdainful eye. He asks the scrub nurse if these are really his glove size. She says that they are his size 8. He still is not sure.

He watches the circulator prepping the patient with iodine scrub and iodine solution. He does not like the patient position and tells the circulator that she missed a spot with the iodine prep. As the drapes are being placed on the patient, he says that he needs another drape. It is not on the back table, the circulator will have to get one from the supply shelf. Now he is annoyed. He asks why the drape was not opened and on the back table before he entered the room. He says that he always uses that extra drape. The circulator is scrambling to get the drape, open it, and hand it to the scrub nurse. The surgeon is waiting impatiently.

The patient is now draped and ready for surgery. The surgeon is at the table and looking for the overhead lights. They are not in the right position. He cannot touch them to put the sterile light-handle covers in place since he is sterile. The circulator adjusts them where he wants them. He gets the covers on and cannot get the lights exactly where he wants. He blames the circulator.

As the procedure starts, he complains that it is too hot in the room. He says that he is perspiring and needs the scrub to wipe his forehead with a towel. He asks again when she is going to cool down the room. He repeats that he is burning up.

The surgeon is ready to begin the procedure. The circulating nurse calls a time-out. The surgeon curses under his breath. It is mandatory that before a surgical procedure starts that the OR team call a time-out to ensure that they have the right patient, the right procedure, and all pertinent information regarding the patient. After reviewing the information, the circulator asks if everyone is in agreement. Everyone says yes. The surgeon turns to the circulator and asks in a sarcastic voice if he may start the procedure.

He starts his incision and tells the anesthetist that the patient is moving. He tells the anesthetist to give him more medication. Oh, and the room is still too hot. He asks what the temperature is in the room. He says that he cannot see. He says that the OR lights need to be turned up. The circulator says that they are all the way up. He shakes his head in disagreement.

While the surgeon is making an incision, the scrub nurse reaches for the next instrument that he will use.

She has anticipated his next procedural step and is ready to hand him what he needs. He criticizes her effort and tells her that he will tell her what he will use and when he will need it. The scrub shakes her head and rolls her eyes. He then asks for the exact instrument that she had in her hand.

The procedure started only fifteen minutes ago, and surgeon has complained about everything. This behavior will continue for the remainder of the procedure. It will make the atmosphere in the room tense. If any of the OR nursing staff brings up a topic for casual conversation, they do it at their own peril. Regardless of the topic, this surgeon will find a way to voice displeasure and disagreement.

The New-Toy Surgeon

These surgeons love new technology and new instruments. To their credit, they are thought leaders. They will champion new products and will pursue their implementation. They will do this for two reasons: they really want to use the newest, best available products, and they really want to get their way. They are rarely concerned about the price.

Surgical salespeople love these surgeons. They are the first surgeons that are pursued for support. Because these surgeons usually perform a high volume of procedures, they have a strong voice in the OR. The OR directors know who these surgeons are also. They are a nightmare for them and their budgets. When the OR director balks at the cost of what the surgeons want, they will band together and meet with the administrator of the hospital. They will ask the administrator to purchase the new equipment and threaten to schedule their procedures at other hospitals if they cannot have the necessary technology. The administrator usually concedes to their wish.

These surgeons cost the OR a lot of money. Quite often, the technology they want is unnecessary or the payback for it is slow or impossible to recover.

I remember when surgical lasers first became popular. The new-toy surgeons had to have them. They asked their administrators to spend hundreds of thousands of dollars to obtain several types of lasers, promising that they would be used in every type of surgery. Further, they would be a grand public relations campaign for their facilities. Once the newness wore off, surgeons found that lasers were limited. Fewer and fewer procedures were performed with them. Today, lasers are used mainly in eye surgery, where they have a vital role. Unfortunately, most lasers sit in OR storage rooms, where they collect dust.

Surgical robots are the new lasers in terms of the latest high-priced technology. Robots cost between $1 and $2 million. The price varies depending on the extras that you order. The new-toy surgeons are ecstatic to learn how to use the robots and become certified for use in their hospitals. Hospitals are conceding to the desire of surgeons to purchase these surgical monsters because they are also a great public relations tool. This has made the public believe that their surgery needs to be performed with a robot.

Robotic surgery comes at an extreme cost. Robots are not only expensive to buy, they are expensive to set up and operate. There is a reimbursement code for use of the robot. However, it is estimated that just to set up the robot for a procedure, the cost is between $1,500 and $2,500. The prices of instrument arms for the robot vary, depending on the type of procedure. But there will be three to five arms per procedure, and that will cost thousands of dollars also. The surgery has not started and the cost is already approaching $5,000.

I have heard experienced surgeons laugh when you ask them about robotic surgery. They think that robots are overpriced and unnecessary. A certified surgeon will perform a procedure without a robot, provide the same clinical results, and will do it for less money.

The new-toy surgeon has a problem with knowing and accepting the difference between needs and wants. Living within a budget should be the same in the health-care field as it is in our individual lives. We all want more than we really need, and it is easier to justify if it is not coming out of our own pockets. The key is accepting the reality of what we are able to afford and not going beyond.

Once the newness wears off, and hospitals get a grip on the excessive cost factors, numerous robots may find themselves alongside the lasers in the OR storage rooms collecting dust.

The Leave-Me-Alone Surgeon

The leave-me-alone surgeons are a no-BS type. They do not complain about not having the latest technology. They do not have huge egos or care to demean and belittle the OR staff. They just want to do their work and be left alone in privacy. In fact, as they walk the halls of the OR, you will see a smile on their faces and never hear a word from them.

They are quiet and unobtrusive. They are usually caring and compassionate surgeons who are skilled and do not need attention and adulation. They are not likely to initiate you in conversation but are always pleasant to you if you engage them. They may not speak much, but they know everything that is happening around them.

OR nurses and scrubs love to work their rooms. During the case, these surgeons are very hands-on before and after the surgery. They will help the nurses with every aspect of patient preparation, positioning, and handling before the procedure. They will also help transfer the patient to the stretcher and often follow the patient to postop care after the procedure.

These surgeons treat the OR team with respect and show common courtesy. They will never make an issue or throw a tantrum if an instrument or accessory is not available. They will make use of what is available in a pleasant, modest, and unassuming way. If a situation becomes tense, they will never lose their composure or raise their voice. They will simply proceed with a calm disposition and demeanor.

I have never seen this type of surgeon say a disparaging word, curse word, or negative thing about anyone or anything. These surgeons are the cornerstones of their profession.

The Humanitarians

The humanitarians are dearly loved and respected. They should be. They are the surgeons who do good works and deeds for those who are in desperate need.

Humanitarians are very friendly and approachable. They have a gracious manner whether in the operating room, the hospital, or their offices. They would never ask that a salesperson or company provide lunches or meals for their staffs. They treat everyone with a genuine warmth and gratitude and are always available.

Humanitarians are usually the better surgeons in the OR. They do not have grandiose egos and seem to be comfortable with themselves. They are usually very interested and willing to try new technology, instruments, and equipment. However, they have a keen interest in cost savings. They would never try to procure products for their personal use that are more expensive. With one exception, the product would have to exhibit a definite advantage and substantially improve patient care. They have a discerning eye for this and have the ability to see how new technology that appears to cost more up-front could actually save money if it offers multiple crossover uses.

A character quality these surgeons have separates them from the rest of their colleagues—total love and devotion for their fellow man. What they do is pro bono for the poor and indigent in America and abroad in third-world countries.

They plan mission trips through their offices or the hospitals where they work. They have their personal nurses call surgical salespeople to ask for surgical supplies that will be used on their trips. They acquire a full array of supplies that will allow them to construct a regular operating room. These supplies are given, at no charge, by surgical corporations. It is one of the few good things that corporations do.

The mission trips may be sponsored through a religious order, a church, a hospital, or a university. The surgeons may also sponsor trips themselves. Regardless of how they are funded, they volunteer their time and talents, free of charge, to help improve people's lives. They also have a team of OR nurses and scrubs that travel with them. These nurses and scrubs also volunteer their time and work out of kindness. Typically, they use their vacation time from the hospital to make these trips.

Most of these missions are to third-world countries where people do not have plumbing or running water. The patients that they treat have serious conditions, and many have never seen a doctor. The surgeons and their team will live in temporary tents or Quonset huts under very stark living conditions.

They will perform surgery with some of the more rudimentary pieces of surgical equipment and products. But they and their OR teams are quite resourceful. Their experiences and skills have taught them how to adapt to any situation and circumstance while still providing the finest in patient care.

The length and regularity of these trips vary. I know of some surgeons and OR teams who make two or three mission trips each year. Each trip lasts a week, and sometimes they are in surgery up to sixteen hours a day.

The giving of themselves to others is deeply rooted in the humanitarian's DNA. They do not do it for glamour or notoriety. It is who they are. There is honor in being humble and giving. The humanitarians are honorable and have the character to live their lives according to the oath and pledge that they made.

They are true surgeons.

Chapter 6 Endnotes:

1. "Surgeon: Career Summary and Required Education," Education Portal, December 31, 2012, http://education-portal.com/articles/Surgeon_Career_Summary_and_Required_Education.html.
2. Alex Macario, "What does one minute of operating room time cost?," *Journal of Clinical Anesthesia* 22 (2010), 233–36, http://ether.stanford.edu/asc/documents.management2.pdf.

Chapter 7
What to Do If You Need Surgery

Do Your Research

You visit your doctor. It may be for a regular appointment. It may be that you have not been feeling well, and you have some persistent symptoms. You tell him or her how you have been feeling and about any unusual conditions. During an examination, your doctor tells you that he or she needs to runs some tests. You ask why. Your doctor says that they are simply routine and not to worry. You suddenly feel flush, and anxiety starts to encompass you. I know the feeling. I have been through this before. And so have millions of people. It is not time to panic. It is time to go to work.

When your doctor says that you need tests, it is important to start asking questions. You will want to know why the tests are being run. What potential diagnoses are of concern? Have your doctor write down for you every pertinent piece of information with the clinical name of each possible condition. Do not rely on your memory. At the present time, you are in a stressed state. You will not remember everything when you return home. And when you return home, you will want to go to your computer and do research on every potential diagnosis that your doctor wrote down for you. Print out copies of this information. Study the information, and take it with you when you have your tests performed.

Your symptoms or conditions will determine where the doctor will send you. You may be sent to a technician for lab tests, blood work, an MRI, or x-rays. If this is the situation, the results will be sent to your doctor. And you will need to have a follow-up visit with him to discuss your results. You may want to question the technician performing your tests about your situation, but he or she is not allowed to discuss your condition or symptoms with you. Only your doctor may.

Based on the test results, your doctor may be able to control or resolve your condition with medicine or therapy. If so, that is a preferable route and is one that should lower your anxiety. But still ask questions. Review the information that you gathered from the computer with your doctor. He or she should have a multitude of information to share with you about your diagnosis, the method of treatment designed for you, and the expected short- and long-term recovery prognosis. Continue to educate yourself about your situation and obey the instructions given by your doctor.

You may also be sent to see another doctor or specialist for more specific work or invasive types of testing. If this is the case, discuss your concerns and worries about what may be happening to you with that doctor. Review with him or her the information that you obtained. Take as much time as needed to have your questions answered. It is your health, and you have the right to know. If you think that this doctor is not answering questions to your satisfaction or meeting your needs, find another doctor.

After the specialist runs his or her series of tests, you will have a follow-up visit with the specialist or your regular doctor to discuss the findings. This is when you may hear those dreaded words that surgery is required. Do not let fear overcome you. Take a deep breath, and try to relax.

If you follow up with the specialist who ran your tests, and he or she is a surgeon, he or she will want to operate. The specialist will ask if you want to schedule a procedure. Do not immediately say yes, unless he or she says that it is an emergency situation. Even then, you will want to know what is meant by emergency. Ask the specialist if you have enough time to see other doctors for their opinions. Several conditions require immediate emergency surgery. If the specialist says that you have no time to wait, follow this advice.

If the specialist says that you have time to consider and seek other opinions, then your real work begins. There are several suggested areas that you need to study before making an informed decision. Once you have gained the necessary knowledge, you will be confident, relaxed, and ready to face the challenge of surgery.

The first thing to do is schedule a revisit with your regular doctor. He or she should anticipate that you have more questions. Ask for more advice about your condition. Ask your regular doctor if he or she would have the surgery if he or she had the same condition. And, more specifically, who would your doctor have operate on him or her? Tell your doctor that you want the names of three surgeons, in order of preference, who would do his or her surgery.

This is important. Quite often, doctors will suggest friends that may belong to the same country club, were medical school classmates, or are associates at the hospitals where they practice. And the doctor may think that any one of them is okay for you. They may be friends, associates, or colleagues of your regular doctor, but your regular doctor may want someone else to do his or her surgery.

Once you have the names of the surgeons, go back to your computer and start doing background checks. Find out as much information as possible about them. You need to know where they went to medical school, their degrees and specialties, how long they have been in practice, and what hospitals have granted them surgical privileges. This will make a great difference in your comfort level.

The background check should also include research for any malpractice lawsuits that have been filed against them. This is information that will not be published by any medical association or hospital. However, most states have a web address that you will be able to access for this type of information. This address will show any litigation that has been taken against an individual in the last five years. Simply enter the surgeon's name. The site will show everything from a traffic ticket and divorce judgments to major lawsuits.

After you have done the investigatory work on your potential surgeons, you need to find a surgical nurse with whom to speak. If you have a nurse friend, ask him or her if he or she would find a surgical nurse who would be willing to speak to you about your surgery. It would really be beneficial if you could speak to one of the surgical nurses who work at the hospitals where your potential surgeons operate.

When you talk to the surgical nurse, do not mention any names. Tell him or her that you are going to have surgery and you believe that the surgery is to be scheduled at his or her hospital. Inform the nurse about your condition and ask for the names of several surgeons he or she would want doing that type of surgery on him or her. If the nurse mentions the name of one of your surgeons, you know that you would be in good hands. If he or she mentions another few names, you may want to go back and reconsider your choices. The nurses who work with the surgeons know everything about them. They know their surgical skills, their attitude under stress, and their bedside manner with patients.

Once you have made your choice of a surgeon, schedule an appointment. You will want to discuss your condition and see if there are any alternatives to having this surgery. Ask about how the surgery will be performed. Discuss the potential risks and complications that may be associated with your particular type of surgery. Ask the surgeon if he or she would have surgery if he or she had this condition. Ask the surgeon how many times he or she has performed this type of surgery.

Get a personal feel for the doctor. Notice whether the doctor takes time to talk to you and does not make you feel rushed. Notice if he or she talks to you in a condescending or patronizing manner. And, lastly, ask the doctor in which hospital he prefers to work. It is important that the surgeon feels completely at ease when doing your surgery. Surgeons know where the better OR surgical teams are. It is usually where they do the majority of their surgery.

Several years ago, I was informed that I needed surgery. I visited a surgeon who was a friend of mine. He and I had been classmates since our middle school days. I knew that he was one of the top-rated surgeons in his specialty because I had done my research. Even though we were friends, I would not have chosen him if I had not known of his expertise. He is a wonderful man and an excellent surgeon. So I had complete confidence about him performing my surgery.

I scheduled an appointment with him to have a few questions answered. I told him that I knew of his privileges at several hospitals. I asked him where he would prefer to work. He said that all of the hospital ORs where he worked were top facilities. However, he said that the anesthesia team at one particular hospital was the best of all. Without saying a negative word about any of the hospitals, he shared with me a very important piece of information. I knew where I wanted to have my surgery. His recommendation was taken. My surgery went smoothly, and I made a complete recovery.

Because I took this approach, I felt empowered about the decisions that I made. I captured a confidence level that helped allay my fears and anxiety. And I felt like my association with my surgeon was more of a partnership.

When you schedule the procedure with your surgeon, there will be many forms to read and sign. *Please read them thoroughly.* Ask questions. Do not sign anything until you have a full understanding and agree to what is in the forms. If there is something in the form that you do not agree with, discuss it with the surgeon. Do not be hesitant to tell him or her exactly what you will and will not accept. The surgeon is in charge of the room during surgery. But you have the ability to make certain requests before he or she operates on you. The surgeon is required to follow those requests.

The surgeon performing your surgery is called the attending surgeon. He or she is the doctor who makes all decisions during the procedure. He or she may also have an assistant surgeon and a physician's assistant. Nurses and scrubs will assist. This is normal protocol. They are needed to perform surgery. You want them to be in the room.

There may also be other medical personnel in the

room. You have the right to include or exclude them from your procedure. If there are residents in the room, tell your surgeon that they will only observe or hold instruments. If there are fellows present, it is perfectly all right for them to assist in the procedure. They are qualified surgeons who are doing a fellowship to increase their skills in a specialty.

Surgeons allow surgical salespeople in the OR when they use a new instrument or try a new type of technology. It is usually stated in the surgical forms for you to sign that you will allow other nonmedical personnel in the room and that your surgeon may determine the use of any instrumentation as he or she deems necessary. You have the right to determine if they may be present and if any new device is to be used on you.

I recommend that you tell your surgeon that you do not want any new instruments used on you for your procedure or salespeople involved in your procedure. You do not know the OR skill level of the salesperson. You also do not know how long the new instrument has been on the market and whether it is trustworthy. Inform your surgeon that you want him or her to do the procedure the way that he or she normally performs it.

There are two exceptions to this opinion. If you are having hip, knee, or total joint replacement, you will want to have the salesperson present. The orthopedic representatives are very well qualified and are an asset. They will offer valuable suggestions for your surgeon to consider. The same is true of salespeople who work with neurosurgeons. They are quite capable and are beneficial to your surgeon.

Either a certified registered nurse anesthetist or anesthesiologist is well qualified to administer anesthesia. However, be sure to tell your surgeon that he or she make three requests from anesthesia: first, that they keep their masks on at all times; second, that they do not play any word games, puzzles, number games, or play with their cell phones while they are monitoring and delivering your anesthesia; and third, that they do not have coffee or drinks in the OR during your procedure. I have the highest respect for their professional abilities and capabilities. I do not accept or appreciate some of their behaviors during surgery.

The thought of having surgery can overwhelm you. To go through the process without any knowledge of how to proceed or what to do is not necessary. Many valuable resources are available to help educate yourself and raise your level of understanding of your options. You do not have to go through it alone. Use family and friends for their support. They may have experience that is beneficial to you.

I hope that the opinions and suggestions that I have made help you along your surgical journey. You are in control. You have the right to decide how, when, where and who will perform your surgery. Make your own decisions with the help of your surgeon. You will find the experience to be successful and rewarding.

Chapter 8
Memories from the Past

Surgeons Doing What They Do

The following stories are fictional depictions of surgeons, nurses, and real-life surgical situations. Any names that I may use are not real. Any attempt to relate them to any specific individual or specific surgical procedure would be an act of pure folly. I would prefer to call it an act of mental masturbation. These are vivid and indelible memories from my past. Or could they have been dreams? It is too difficult to remember.

I Don't Want Lip Service

I remember conducting an evaluation in the operating room suite of a large nonprofit hospital. The OR was budgeted to purchase fifteen pieces of energy-based equipment, one piece for each room. Fifteen pieces of equipment would be a large purchase and would provide me with a substantial commission. Three companies were vying for the business. Quotes were submitted and evaluation approval was given to each manufacturer.

Each company was given a week for its equipment to be brought into the OR for the surgical staff, surgeons, and nurses to evaluate in clinical situations. Evaluation forms would be completed by each surgeon and nurse for every procedure in which they participated. The staff input is always instrumental in all decisions on equipment. Their decision is usually made and based on which product offers any clinical superiority and has the best price. However, I have found that being the last company in line for evaluation works to your advantage. The last memory is the lasting memory. I was excited that I was the final company to be evaluated.

I brought three pieces of equipment to the hospital. They would need to be inspected and tested for safety before taking them to the OR. After safety inspection, I conducted an in-service with the OR nursing staff early on a Monday morning. It went very well. The nursing staff gave a lot of positive feedback and showed interest in the technology that my company had to offer.

I needed to do clinical work with all of the different services: general, neurosurgery, orthopedics, gynecology, plastics, urology, ENT, and cardiothoracic. It is crucial to work with as many surgeons as possible in clinical procedures. You do not want to overlook any doctor. The one that you overlook may take offense, and that one surgeon might have the greatest influence in the decision-making process.

Monday through Thursday, the evaluation went incredibly well. I had worked with most of the influential surgeons. I received positive evaluations from every surgeon, most of whom recommended purchasing my surgical equipment over my competition. The nursing staff was also in my favor. They thought that my equipment was easier to use than my competitors'. Most importantly, they knew that the surgeons were pleased. When the surgeons are pleased, the nurses are pleased.

Friday was to be my last day of clinical trials. I was scheduled to work with an otolaryngologist. He had several tonsil and adenoid procedures to perform. I introduced myself to the surgeon at the scrub sink before the procedure to see if he had any questions about my equipment. He said that he did not. But he said that he was going to try a new technique for his procedures that he learned at a training course. The technique incorporated the use of bipolar energy instead of using traditional monopolar energy. I told him that I was interested in understanding this approach and observing.

The first T and A was to be performed on a seven-year-old boy. The equipment was set up, and the instruments were connected to the energy source. The procedure began. He used cold steel dissection to completely remove the tonsil and then reached for the bipolar forceps to coagulate the tonsil bed. He placed the forceps in the boy's mouth and activated the instrument with the footswitch. One of the tongs of the forceps touched the boy's lip. He quickly stopped and yelled, "Damn it! Your equipment just gave this boy a third-degree burn on his lip." He said to get my equipment out of the OR. He was pissed. The nurses moved quickly to disconnect my generator and replace it with their regular one.

I looked at the forceps that he was using and noticed that they were not insulated. Using an uninsulated instrument with electrical equipment may cause burns on unintended tissue. It is extremely risky and ill advised, at best. I asked him why he would use forceps that were not insulated. He looked at me in surprise. He said that he was not aware that they were uninsulated. At that point, the scrub nurse said, "Doctor, you know that those forceps are not insulated. You have used them before in other procedures."

The surgeon told the circulating nurse to get the OR director in the room immediately. He told me to leave the OR immediately. I went to the nurses' lounge to wait. This was not a pleasant scenario. A patient receiving a surgical burn could mean a lawsuit. This situation would need to be handled in a delicate way. I was eager to speak with the OR director and the surgeon when the procedure was over.

Within minutes, the OR director met with me in the lounge. She said that the evaluation was over and that I should leave the hospital. I was not to take the piece of equipment that was used in the T and A with me.

She said that it would be confiscated and quarantined until it was determined if there would be any legal action from the burn on the patient. I tried to engage her in conversation and discuss with her why the evaluation was canceled. I also wanted to discuss the burn incident with her. There was no interest on her part to talk. She said that she was not able to discuss the evaluation or the incident that happened.

I was terribly concerned and emotionally deflated. One minute I was conducting a highly successful evaluation with total acceptance by the staff. The next minute the evaluation was being terminated, and I was being asked to leave the hospital. I was most concerned about the young boy with the burn on his lip and if there would be legal action against me and my company.

As I was leaving the OR, I saw the surgeon involved in the incident. I called to him and walked toward him. When he heard his name called, he turned and saw me. He immediately turned his back to me and continued to walk away. I wanted to discuss with him what happened and why. He was refusing to speak with me. He would not even look me in the eye.

I was not awarded the business. It went to one of my competitors. And the reason why? The surgeon made a blatant mistake. He used an instrument where it never should have been used. He later tried to place blame on my equipment, saying that it was not clinically acceptable because it was dangerous. All of the effort that I had put into that evaluation went to waste because a surgeon made a gross error in judgment. And he did not have the moral character to admit it. Instead, he placed blame elsewhere.

This type of behavior from a surgeon occurs all the time. I have seen a lot of mistakes made by surgeons. I have not seen or heard very many apologies or admissions of culpability. They believe that they are always right and can do no wrong.

I met with the director of biomedical engineering for the hospital. Biomedical technicians are the employees who test, check, and repair all hospital equipment. This includes doing safety checks on all evaluation equipment that comes into the hospital. All evaluation equipment must pass inspection before being used in clinical areas. He said that his technician checked my equipment when it came in the hospital, and checked it again after the OR incident. He said that both times, the equipment checked out perfectly. Also, I asked him if he knew about the burn incident in the OR. He stated that he was familiar with the situation. He further mentioned that he could not believe that the surgeon could be so "stupid."

The hospital did not return that piece of equipment to me for over a year. It is my understanding that the hospital and the surgeon agreed to a settlement with the family out of court. That is the usual outcome. Neither the hospital nor the surgeon wants the negative press or public relations fiasco.

I am happy if the family received a settlement. People deserve to be financially compensated when there is a mistake made by a surgeon that has an effect on their health.

The young boy involved in that incident would be a young man now. I hope that he is doing well.

The Case That Went Up in Smoke

During surgery certain electrical devices produce smoke when they are used on human tissue. This smoke, or smoke plume, as it is called, has been carefully studied for several years. The most recent studies show that this smoke plume contains dozens of known toxic, hazardous, carcinogenic, and infectious agents. It is now classified as a hazardous material. Some federal agency laws recommend that it be suctioned away from the OR surgical table with smoke evacuation devices that have high-grade filters. This is done to protect the nurses and surgeons from breathing and ingesting it. Albeit, there are still surgeons who do not believe that this smoke is hazardous.

Most surgeons only work two or three days a week in the OR and during that time only perform a few surgeries. They are not daily and constantly in this toxic, smoke-filled environment. But OR nurses work every day in that environment. The surgical masks that are worn during surgery do not have the capability to filter this smoke plume. So they breathe and consume this smoke all day. Estimates say burning one gram of tissue smoke may release the same components as three to six cigarettes.[1] During an average working day, the OR nurses breathe in many times this amount. And there are increasing numbers of nurses who have chronic illnesses due to surgical smoke. In fact, some statistics show that OR nurses have at least twice the chance of acquiring illnesses related to chronic obstructive pulmonary disease, or COPD, as the general public.[2]

A hospital called me to schedule an evaluation of my surgical equipment that included a smoke evacuation system. The OR nursing administration was eager to comply with the new federal standards and to purchase several smoke evacuation systems that could protect the health and safety of their nurses and doctors.

I arrived at the hospital early in the morning, changed into surgical attire and went to the nurses' lounge to in-service the energy equipment and smoke system. The staff was excited that I was there and relieved to know that their hospital cared enough about their health to initiate such a program.

I reviewed the surgery schedule for the day with the OR nurse educator. We targeted surgical cases that would normally produce the most smoke. Those cases would be the biggest test for the smoke evacuation system. They would also make the greatest impression on the staff.

The first two procedures that I worked went well. The nurses were very receptive and were able to gently urge the surgeons to evaluate the systems. The surgeons immediately noticed the improved atmosphere and lack of smoke plume. I discussed the potential hazards of surgical smoke with them and gave them several white papers to review. Later, they agreed to support implementation of the systems.

My third case was the removal of a melanoma from the anterior thigh of a middle-aged woman. I would be working with a different surgeon. I met with the nurses before the procedure as they were setting up the room. The patient and surgeon had not arrived yet. The nurses were particularly interested in using the smoke evacuator for this procedure. The lesion was rather large, and this surgeon liked to use higher settings on the equipment, which meant that there would be a higher level of smoke. The nurses did not like the idea of breathing smoke from a melanoma lesion.

I met the surgeon as he approached the scrub sink. I introduced myself and explained why I was there. I reviewed with him the data on surgical smoke and asked his permission to set up my energy equipment and smoke evacuation system for his case. He said that he would be interested in evaluating my energy source, but he said that he would not be using the smoke evacuator. I asked him why. He said that he did not believe all of that crap about surgical smoke being hazardous. I then asked him if he smoked cigarettes, cigars, or pipes. He said no, and that smoking is hazardous to your health. I told him that if he is not using smoke evacuation in his surgical procedures, then he and all of his nurses are smoking. He just shook his head and walked to the OR door.

As he walked into the room, he asked me if I was coming in to observe. I said not unless he would use the smoke evacuator. He laughed and walked toward the OR table. The door closed behind him. As he was gowning, I heard the nurses start to discuss the smoke evacuation system with him. He was not pleased with what they were saying and quickly began chastising them in a loud voice. They looked bewildered. I watched the case from the hallway. There was smoke everywhere. None of the nurses were smiling or talking.

After the procedure I spoke with the nurses who worked the room. They were visibly upset with him. And they really went off on him. They said that he was a pain to work with in the OR, that he was very stubborn and very arrogant, and that he thought he was an expert on everything. They called it the God syndrome. No matter what you do, it will be wrong, and he will attempt to correct you. That sounded familiar to me. They were also worried about his opposition to using smoke evacuation products. He performed a lot of procedures and was very influential in the OR. They hoped that he would not thwart their efforts to acquire the smoke evacuation systems.

The rest of the evaluation went well. The nurses and surgeons were receptive and pleased to have a "breath of fresh air" in the OR. They did not have to breathe the suffocating and toxic surgical smoke.

I received an order for ten energy units and ten smoke evacuation systems several weeks later. It was very rewarding. It made me feel that I was helping to improve the working environment for the OR staff.

The nurses were able to get what they needed for their safety in spite of that one obstinate surgeon. I would like to think that even if he did not believe that surgical smoke is dangerous to your health, he did not interfere with the staff getting what they believed they needed for their safety.

That incident happened more than five years ago. The nursing staff uses the smoke evacuation systems on almost every procedure, and they are very pleased with them. I know, to this day, that surgeon has never used the smoke evacuators. I am sure that he never will.

If You Can't Catch, Don't Pitch

Laparoscopy is one of the more popular surgical techniques used today. It may be used for many types of surgical procedures. It may help save OR time and money, is less stressful, and shortens the full recovery time for the patient. Most surgeons would prefer to perform laparoscopic surgery when possible, especially when it comes to saving time. Whenever possible, surgeons are interested in saving time.

The instruments used in laparoscopic surgery are different than the ones used for open procedures. Laparoscopic instruments have a longer shaft and are smaller in diameter. This design enables them to be passed through trocars. A trocar is a cylindrical cannula that is placed in a cavity of the surgical patient.

A surgeon may place anywhere from two to five trocars in a patient, depending on the type of procedure. They are only 5 mm, 10 mm, or 12 mm in diameter, so the patient would only have a few small incisions and not one large incision. This allows for a faster recovery.

One type of laparoscopic instrument that is used in most procedures is a suction coagulator. It will allow for electrosurgical dissection of tissue, coagulation, and fluid irrigation and suction. Many companies market this type of instrument. Most of them have the same basic method of use. However, each company may have some variation in application method or nuance that needs to be understood before using in surgery. The instrument that I sold had a protective sheath that extends over the cutting electrode tip and protects it during irrigation and suction. There is a unique way to extend and retract that sheath that needs to be explained and seen. In other words, the nurses and surgeons needed to be in-serviced.

I was working an evaluation of my suction coagulators in a large hospital. I held an in-service for the nursing staff on the product. It was received well, and I was ready to work the suite. Surgeons will never attend these in-services. Their time is too valuable, or so they think. Usually, I will in-service the surgeon at the scrub sink just before the scheduled surgery. It is common to tell the surgeon who you are, what you have and why it is clinically superior, and ask if there is interest. Also, it is of the utmost importance to ask the surgeon for permission to be in the room during clinical use.

Surgeons are in charge of their OR, and some have egos that can be easily offended.

One of the better procedures for first-time evaluation of a laparoscopic instrument is a laparoscopic cholecystectomy. That is the laparoscopic removal of a gall bladder. During this procedure, there is cutting, coagulating, fluid irrigation, and suction. There was one on the schedule. I went to the room while the nurses were setting up the case and brought my instrument. I told the nurses that I would demonstrate it to the surgeon at the sink and find out if he would agree to use it.

As the surgeon approached the sink, I introduced myself and told him why I was there. I had a sample of the suction irrigator in my hand so that he could hold it and see how it worked as I explained the unique dynamics. He was distant and unfriendly and seemed in a hurry. I began showing him how the hand piece was used, but he was not watching me. He stopped me in midsentence and, in a condescending voice, said, "I know how to work a simple suction irrigator. I have used them before. Just bring it in."

I entered the OR and gave the sterile instrument to the circulator to hand to the scrub nurse for the procedure. The case began, and you could see that the doctor was in a hurry. He was working fast, and there was little or no conversation. That is usually an indication that the nurses are aware that the doctor is not in a good mood. He used my instrument to dissect some adhesions and coagulate some small bleeders and dissect the gall bladder from the liver bed. It worked perfectly. Now, he was at a point in the procedure where he needed the instrument for irrigation and suction. As he tried to extend the protective sheath, he could not get it to work. The scrub tried to show him, but he rebuffed her. I tried to explain to him, but he was in such a hurry and frustrated that he would not listen.

In a fit of frustration, he disconnected the suction and irrigation line on the instrument and threw it at me from the OR field. I heard a gasp from the scrub nurse. The circulator asked him what he thought he was doing. He said that the instrument did not work, and to get him the one that he always uses.

I was wearing latex gloves and tried to catch it. I missed; the instrument landed against my chest. I had blood and body fluid all over my arms and scrub suit. The circulating nurse was embarrassed and apologized to me repeatedly. I said that it was not her fault. You could have cut the mood in that room with a knife. There was not one sound.

I needed to leave the room, wash off, and change my scrub suit. But before I left the room, I needed to know if the instrument was broken. If it was, I owed the surgeon an apology. I tried to work the instrument. I was able to operate all of the functions on the hand piece. It was in perfect working condition.

After changing clothes, I went to the nurses' lounge. My instrument was no longer being used, and I needed to take a break. Some time later, I heard over the intercom a request for me to meet the surgeon outside the room where the case was performed. I met him there, and he apologized to me for his behavior. He asked me to accept his apologies. He said that he had been working late the night before on call and offered a few other excuses. I said that I accepted his apology but not his excuses. I told him that I thought there was no reason for that behavior. He did not like what he heard me say. I could see an arrogant smile return to his face. He turned around and walked away.

This surgeon was wrong for several reasons. Firstly, if he would have listened to me and watched my explanation of how to use the device at the scrub sink, that incident would never have happened. Secondly, that kind of temperament for a surgeon during a procedure could be detrimental to the patient's safety and well-being. And, lastly, by subjecting me to a person's bodily fluids, I could have been at risk of acquiring any blood disorder that the patient might have had.

I never worked with him again.

There Will Be a Test Tomorrow

I believe that salespeople have been maligned for quite some time. The majority are honest, hardworking people who have great respect for their profession and their customers. That is how they achieve trust and earn a lot of money. There are many stories about the lies and half-truths from salespeople's lips. All they do is help to belittle and demean the sales profession. And I do not deny that I have seen and heard some shifty salespeople in the past. However, I have seen shifty people in all aspects of business.

In the surgical sales business, it is quite different. It is not like selling a used car. When asked a question, you tell the truth. Or at least you tell what you know. If you do not know the technical aspects of your product, its clinical capabilities, and the anatomy involved in the procedure in which it is used, a surgeon will know it in a heartbeat.

And then you will lose all credibility.

I was working a surgical trade show a number of years ago. This particular national show attracts thousands of surgeons from all over the world. Every medical manufacturer from all over the world attends also. There are working product displays set up by the manufacturers to show surgeons the latest technology. And there are plenty of salespeople to greet surgeons, involve them in product demonstrations, and pique their interest to evaluate at their hospital.

I was standing at one corner of my company booth when a surgeon approached and asked about an electrosurgical generator for use in his surgical procedures. He asked some quite specific questions regarding electricity and the RF current used in the equipment. So I began discussing with him current power, wavelength forms, crest factors, peak to peak voltage, controlling voltage release, and isolated circuitry. He then asked about the difference between monopolar and bipolar delivery. I explained it to him.

He then changed his interest to specific settings on the generator and asked what setting he should use in monopolar cut and coagulation if he was doing a circumcision. I replied that I believed only bipolar coagulation current was indicated for a circumcision, not monopolar, and that monopolar usage was contraindicative in that procedure. He smiled and said, "I know that; I wanted to see if you did."

The surgeon agreed to evaluate the equipment, and I worked with him one week later. During one procedure he said that he was impressed with my knowledge of my product and its clinical application. I told him that I was impressed with his knowledge of electricity. I said that most surgeons do not seem that interested in electricity. Their only care is if the generator will cut and coagulate. He said that his bachelor's degree was in electrical engineering. It all made sense. At the medical show, he was testing me to see if I really knew about electricity, energy-based equipment, and their safe application.

He was instrumental in obtaining approval to purchase my generator for his hospital. And he was instrumental in teaching me a lesson. Surgeons are like lawyers; when they ask a question, they already know the answer. Do not ever try to fool them.

Please Do Not Touch

Have you ever told someone not to do something three or four times and then seen them do it anyway? Isn't it frustrating? Imagine that happening with a doctor. Imagine a doctor not listening to explicit instructions, doing the opposite, and damaging a patient's esophagus. Imagine that patient needing emergency surgery to repair the damage. Imagine what would happen to you.

I was working with a group of doctors in the gastroenterology lab. They were evaluating a type of technology that my company sold. This particular technology created coagulation in tissue without contacting or touching the tissue. In fact, contacting or touching tissue with this technology was contraindicative. It is clearly stated in the equipment technical information manual, and by all salespeople working with doctors, to not touch tissue when using this technology. And the possible consequences if misused are stated.

My company was given several weeks for the evaluation. This would allow each gastroenterologist enough time to use it in several clinical trials. The doctors in the department were familiar with this technology. They recently completed a trial evaluation with my competitor and were using this technology at other hospitals.

I set up a working display of my equipment in the nurses' lounge and conducted several in-services. The staff could see and operate the device. In the GI lab, doctors visited the working display so that they knew how it functioned and how to use it on a patient.

I in-serviced a doctor and explained the features and benefits of my technology. I also explained why my product was safer and superior to the competition. As always, I emphasized that when using this technology never to touch or contact tissue and what the potential consequences of touching tissue were. She said that she understood.

The doctor said that she had an EGD scheduled that morning and wanted to have the equipment in the room. She thought that she might need to use it with this particular patient. I was somewhat surprised that she would consider using an electrosurgical device for an EGD. I have found that most doctors are hesitant to use equipment that would conduct electricity in the esophagus. But she was the doctor. I assumed that she knew what she was doing.

I took the equipment to her room. The EGD was to be performed on a middle-aged man. He complained of a cough and said he had blood in his mucous. The doctor would place a scope in his mouth and extend it down his esophagus and into his stomach. This would enable her to view his entire upper GI tract.

During examination with the scope, the doctor discovered that the man had a small tear in his esophagus that was bleeding. She decided that she would need my equipment. I connected a probe to the machine and discussed with the doctor about inserting it in the scope and how to maneuver the probe to ablate the tissue and stop the bleeding. I told her to maintain a distance of one centimeter from the tissue at all times, especially during activation to avoid complications.

When she arrived at the area that she wanted to treat, I instructed her again how it should be operated and reminded her to maintain a one-centimeter distance from the tissue before and after activation. The doctor laid the probe against the man's esophagus and activated the probe. As she was activating, I told her to remove the probe from the tissue. It was too late. The effect of the probe lying on the tissue caused a huge divot in the lining of his esophagus.

The bleeding stopped, but I heard the circulating nurse say that the divot was pretty severe. The doctor tried to downplay the situation and said that everything was fine. But I knew what the circulating nurse was saying. It was not okay. I could not believe it when the doctor said that she was finished. She thanked me for my support and said that she liked the clinical effect from my equipment. I left the procedure room. I had an uneasy feeling. I worked the rest of the day without monitoring any other procedures.

I returned to the GI Lab the following morning to continue the evaluation. As I walked into the department, I was greeted by a nurse who said that I needed to see the director of the department. I did not have a good feeling. I knew that something was wrong.

The director told me that the man with the esophageal tear needed emergency surgery last night to correct the divot created during his procedure. And the doctor was blaming me and my company for the problem. I was shocked. The director said that the evaluation was being terminated. The hospital would be in contact with my company.

When a problem like this occurs, an incident report needs to be filed with your company within twenty-four hours of notification of the incident. This is required by the federal government. I completed my report and e-mailed it to my company before the end of that day.

I was able to meet with the doctor who made the mistake. Her disposition had totally changed. She was so nice and gracious when I left the day before. Now she was accusatory and fuming. I reminded her about my suggestions of not touching tissue and the potential complications that could occur. She did not seem to remember. She even suggested that I was making a veiled threat about her proficiency as a doctor. I tried to explain further, but she said that she had nothing more to discuss with me.

I was not going to let this go. I have learned that when you are right, you must defend yourself. I went to the circulating nurse that worked the case with us the day before. He knew about the patient needing follow-up emergency surgery. I told him what the doctor said and what she told the director of the department. I asked him for his help. He remembered me telling the doctor several times to not touch tissue during the procedure and said that he remembered me mentioning that during all of my in-servicing. He said that he would talk to the director of the department.

It is unusual for nurses to go against a doctor's word.

They could lose their jobs. But in this instance, I found out that more than one nurse spoke to the director of the department about my instructions during in-servicing. Whatever was said or done must have worked, because neither I nor my company heard from the hospital. The hospital or doctor never heard from me again, either.

It Is Music to My Ears

In sales, you never know what will be the determining factor in gaining the business. Everyone has different wants and needs. It is the salesperson's job to identify that want or need and try to satisfy it. Sometimes it is quite difficult. Other times it is surprisingly easy. But that is one of the many things that make sales so exciting. It is like trying to solve a puzzle.

I was working an equipment evaluation at a for-profit hospital. There were several companies on contract that the hospital OR would be evaluating, so pricing would be a major issue.

I was making the rounds, working with different surgeons. Everything was running smoothly. I knew who the more influential surgeons were and made arrangements to work with them. The chief of surgery was a general surgeon. He did a lot of work and would have the most say in which company would be awarded the business. I would need to be in his OR for at least two or three days.

I started working with him on a Tuesday. He was a

very likable person and had a low-key personality. He was warm, kind, and liked to listen to music in the OR. He would sing when he heard one of his favorite tunes. I heard the circulating nurse ask him if it was his birthday tomorrow. He said yes. And small talk ensued about his birthday plans with his family and the usual talk of being one year older. I believed him to be my age, so I could identify with the importance of the one-year-older thing.

Then I had an idea. I recently put together a ten-CD collection of all of the music hits from the '60s. That decade of music was popular when I was in high school. He liked music and was my age. I would make a copy of the collection and give it to him as a present on his birthday.

I arrived in surgery the next morning with the CD collection gift-wrapped. I went to his room before surgery and told the circulating nurse what I had done. She said that was great and that he would really appreciate the gift. I waited in the hallway outside his OR; when he arrived I wished him happy birthday and gave him the present. He looked surprised and a little embarrassed. He opened the box and I explained what was inside. He smiled, shook my hand, and thanked me. He was as happy as could be.

He scrubbed at the sink and then entered the OR. The patient was under anesthesia. He gowned and gloved and was ready to work. He told the circulator to put on one of the CDs. As the music began to play, he began to sing at the top of his voice. He was moving to the music. He looked at me and gave me the thumbs-up. He was in heaven. For the rest of the day he sang and moved to the music. When surgery was over for that day, he said that he was forever thankful.

I worked the rest of the week with several other surgeons. The evaluations that I received were okay. According to most of the staff, there was not any real difference between my equipment and that of my competitors. That made me nervous. As a salesperson, you need some kind of perceived advantage or value added, or what is called a competitive edge over the competition, which will make customers want and need your product. This is especially true in price-sensitive situations. I knew that our price was neither the highest nor the lowest. So I did not have price on my side.

The next week, I went to the purchasing office to review the price proposal for the OR equipment with the material manager. During our conversation, he said that he heard about the gift that I had given to the chief of surgery. My heart became lodged in my throat. I thought that he was going to give me a tongue-lashing for trying to bribe a surgeon with a gift. Instead, he asked if it would be any trouble to make him a copy of the CD collection. He even offered to pay for it. I said that it would be no problem, and it would not cost him a cent. It would be my way of thanking him and the hospital for evaluating my equipment.

A few days later, I returned to the purchasing office with the CD collection. The purchasing agent looked through the listing of songs on each one and just shook his head. He smiled and shook my hand. I told him that I was grateful for the opportunity to work with his hospital staff. As I was about to leave, he said that he had something for me. He opened up a notebook on his desk and handed me a purchase order for fifteen surgical systems.

I was pleasantly surprised and felt like a million dollars. That is the way it is with sales. There are incredible highs and lows. I always look back and try to determine what made the difference. Often, I laugh when I realize how easy it was. Sometimes it just means being kind and thoughtful. Other times I am overly stressed because it was so difficult and complicated. During those times, there are no good feelings. Win or lose, you are just happy to have it done.

Thinking back, that was probably the easiest sale that I ever made. Everything flowed smoothly. There were no problems, errors, or malfunction issues. I was eager to fax the order to my company. I arrived home at the end of the day, and as I listened to the fax machine hum, it sounded like music to my ears.

She Was a Crotchety Sort

Medical trade shows or conventions are a lot of work. The days are filled with grueling hours of standing on your feet and trying to keep a smile on your face. Anyone who has worked a trade show knows that they are a necessary evil. They try your patience and endurance, but just one product presentation could initiate a large-scale evaluation, sale, and commission.

I was attending a medical/surgical trade show for operating room nurses as a representative for my company. It was one of the larger yearly nursing trade shows in the United States. Each year, it is held in a different major city. That year it was in New Orleans. The nurse attendees measured in the thousands. Medical/surgical manufacturers and suppliers had display booths to present their products and discuss important nursing issues related to their hospitals and surgeons. This convention lasted four days.

At the end of each working day, the company representatives would return to their hotels. Most companies provided their own individual hospitality suites at their hotel headquarters. These suites were made available to any and all nurses. They were catered and supplied with the most elaborate settings of food and drink imaginable. The amount of money that corporations spend on these types of affairs is mentally overwhelming. I have always wondered how much money is spent on a yearly basis by corporations in the United States for entertainment. Whether it is the medical, industrial, or retail industry, it has to be in the billions of dollars. It must certainly work in helping to obtain business. If it did not work, they would not do it.

The nurses would move from suite to suite, and hotel to hotel, to enjoy the free array of entertainment. They also wanted to see who was having the best party. It was not uncommon for these hospitality suite parties to last well into the early-morning hours. And as the nights grew longer, the types of activities that occurred grew more lurid.

In any working environment, it is essential and wise to watch your behavior. My philosophy has always been to not say or do anything that you could not say or do in front of your mother. It has always seemed to work for me. Companies are always conducting sessions on sexual harassment and are very conscious of what employees are doing and saying at conventions and at regional or national meetings.

The activity that clearly justifies the most scrutiny is alcohol consumption. I have seen more sales careers ruined by alcohol, and by the subsequent bad behavior that follows, than any other reason. Companies know this. They know that one slip by a company representative, even if inadvertent, could cost them millions in a lawsuit.

I was at the company hospitality suite one particular evening. I was mingling with visitors and looking for any nurses from my sales region. These social gatherings are a great way to establish a friendly relationship with your customers in an environment away from their jobs. I had a drink in one hand and a small plate of appetizers in the other. A nurse approached me and said hello. I acknowledged her and introduced myself. I set down my appetizer plate and offered my hand to shake. Instead of reaching to shake my hand, I felt her hand in my groin on my genitals. I was stunned, took a step back, and said excuse me. She took a step forward, still had a hand on my genitals, and said that she wanted to explore a part of my anatomy. As I was telling her that it was not possible, one of the company's senior managers appeared. He asked what was going on. The young lady left quickly.

This manager was irate. He had not seen the whole scenario, only that a woman had me in a compromised position. And, of course, he assumed that I was the one at fault. I tried to explain the situation to him, but he would not listen. He told me that he saw what happened. He stated that he would talk to my immediate sales manager and recommend that I be terminated. I had never felt worse in my life. I was going to lose my job because of the lewd actions of some drunk.

The manager told me to leave the hospitality suite and go directly to my room. He said that I would be meeting with him and my immediate sales manager in the morning. As I was leaving, another senior manager stopped me. He said that he saw everything that transpired. And he said that I was not to blame and did nothing wrong. He said that he would talk to the other senior manager and my immediate sales manager. He assured me that I would not lose my job.

The next morning, I met with the two senior managers and my immediate sales manager. I was pleasantly surprised when the accusing manager apologized for jumping to conclusions about the incident the night before. He said that I did not have to worry about my job. He was made aware of what really happened.

We all stood and shook hands. I thanked him for understanding, and I thanked the other senior manager for giving me the support that saved my career. My immediate sales manager smiled and winked at me.

I will always remember the support that man gave me. He took a chance with his own career to help save mine. That is something that is not often seen in business. Usually it happens the other way. People in the corporate world cannot wait to find a way to eliminate you or take your job. They do it as blood sport while trying to mollify their incredulous insecurities.

As for the intoxicated nurse who almost cost me my job, I am sure that she found what she wanted.

Dr. Nepotism

In every field of business, there are certain sale situations where you will fail to attain the order because of unseen circumstances. Sometimes you work so hard. You plan every step along the way, rethink your approach, and constantly try to foresee anything that could go wrong or arise to thwart your efforts. You strike down every possible objection and negative. And you still lose.

I was involved in a hospital evaluation of surgical equipment. As usual, the hospital called and asked me to participate. Most hospitals need to have three company bids and conduct evaluations with each before giving an award. I had already presented and reviewed my price proposal with the purchasing department. I knew from my conversation with the material manager that the cost of my equipment was appreciably less than the other two manufacturers. I was feeling pretty good.

I was the last of the three companies to be evaluated. The other two companies were found to be clinically acceptable to the surgeons and nurses. I had no doubt that my equipment would be found acceptable also. Several of the surgeons in this hospital were using my equipment at other facilities and were pleased with it. I was feeling a guarded sense of confidence. I thought that it was about a 90 percent sure thing.

I worked the OR evaluation for one full week. I covered every service and received favorable evaluation forms from every nurse and almost every doctor. There was only one exception. One surgeon was not pleased with the thought of evaluating the equipment, and he was very surly to me! Several times during the evaluation period, I extended to him the opportunity to trial during a procedure. Every time, he would turn me down.

One morning, I approached him to discuss the trial. He would not take the time to stand still and speak with me. He walked away, with his back to me, as I followed behind and tried to engage him in conversation. He would not address me face to face. I asked him if he had any concerns about evaluating, or if I had done anything to offend him. He said no. However, I knew that something was wrong.

I still felt pretty good about my chances; 100 percent of the nurses found the product clinically acceptable.

Nineteen out of twenty surgeons found it favorable. My price was the lowest. What could possibly go wrong?

Well, I did not get the business. It was awarded to the company that had the highest bid. There was a secret that I did not know. The surgeon who would not even consider my equipment had a nephew that was the sales representative for the company that won the business. That surgeon had talked to the other surgeons and encouraged them to support his nephew.

I found out what really happened from one of the OR nurses. She said that no one was supposed to talk about the decision. I went to the OR director and the material manager to discuss and complain. I asked them to explain to me what happened. They said that it was out of their hands. The surgeons made the decision. Conveniently, neither of them made mention of the surgeon and his nephew.

I was extremely depressed and dumbfounded. But I quickly regained my composure and game face. You learn in sales to not take things personally. And you do not dwell on lost sales. You have to be positive and move on to the next opportunity.

Ethics, Morals, and Surgery

When you work as a surgical salesperson, you enter the operating room every day not knowing what will be on the schedule. After arriving and changing into OR attire, you go to the surgery board to see what the day has to offer. Depending on the type of hospital, there will be limited or extended types of procedures. Usually, the larger the hospital, the more diverse types of procedures you will have an opportunity to work.

During my career, I have observed and worked in thousands of different surgical procedures. I have seen some so often that if I had a nickel for each time, I would be a rich man. Others are rarely performed, and to see them is left to timing and chance. When you do find one of the rare ones, it can be a wonderful learning experience. If you know the surgeon, he/she usually will allow you to observe and may discuss the step-by-step process. Surgeons love to teach.

I was working an equipment evaluation in a large outpatient surgery center not associated with any hospital. This facility was part of a for-profit system. Thirty operating rooms were in this center. It was the largest one that I have visited.

One morning, I arrived at the surgery center, changed my clothes, and went to the surgery board. What I saw was incredulous to me. On the schedule was a sexual reassignment procedure—a sex change procedure. I was surprised beyond belief and was excited. I was surprised because this was an outpatient surgery center. A procedure of this nature is long and involved. It requires a team of several different types of surgeons. Each would perform his or her specialty portion of the operation. From what I understood, this type of surgery would require at least an overnight stay. Most patients in surgery centers are sent home the same day. However, this facility did have overnight-stay capabilities. And I was excited because in all my years of working in the operating room, this was the one procedure that I had never observed.

My eyes quickly scanned the surgery board to the name of the surgeon who would be leading the team. I knew him! I had worked with him in two other hospitals. He was a very experienced and excellent surgeon. He had a great disposition, was very gracious, and was the kind of surgeon with whom nurses want to work.

I waited outside of the OR where the procedure was scheduled. When I saw the surgeon, I approached him and said hello. He remembered me and called me by name. I engaged him in the usual small talk. And then I asked him a favor. I told him that I had never seen a sex change procedure and asked him if I might observe. He said that he would love to have me there.

There was talk among the nurses about that procedure earlier in the morning. This was the late '80s. And, although this type of procedure was not new to the surgery world, it was one that still stirred much controversy. Several of the nurses refused to work the case. And there were raised voices and bickering back and forth in relation to the ethics and morals involved. I kept my mouth shut. I knew better than to get involved.

There were nurses who finally agreed to do the procedure. They set up the room and brought in the patient. I talked with the lead surgeon at the sink and thanked him for this opportunity. He said that he would be happy to explain the process if I was interested. I said that I would be thrilled to learn. We entered the room, and I established myself out of the way and against a wall.

The surgery lasted the entire day, with several changes in the nursing team and the surgeon in charge. I was in awe, as were several of the nurses. They had never been involved in a case like this before. There were many questions asked about the surgery and, of course, the ethics and morals of doing this. The expertise and hand skills of the surgeons were amazing. The conversation was stimulating and insightful.

There was one particular portion of the room conversation that I found fascinating. The lead surgeon was discussing the process that surgery candidates have to go through before they finally qualify for the procedure. And then he asked a question. He asked, "Do you know what the most disturbing thing about performing this surgery is for me?" I said no. He said that about 40 percent of the patients who have a sex change procedure will want to return to their original sex in about four years. I was taken aback.

I said that I had a question for him. He said that he knew what the question was. He said that I was going to ask him why, then, would he do the surgery. I told him that he was correct. He said that it was not his position to judge or inject his views on ethics and morals. He explained how many of these people have a great amount of personal agony and anguish in their lives.

He was merely providing a service to help improve the quality of this patient's life and grant his wish. Now I understood from a totally different perspective.

Surgical salespeople do not see a person during an operation. The patient is totally draped and covered. We never know them as people, know their names, or have the ability to find how their recoveries progress. Often, I think back on a certain difficult or traumatic procedure and wonder how the patient recovered. We may not know the patients as people, but some of these cases tear at our emotions and sense of humanity. It is impossible to not have sympathy and feelings for what some surgical patients have to endure.

In this particular case, I hope that this person is at peace, has found comfort and happiness, and enjoys a loving support system of family and friends.

Vive La France!

There are times when the most bizarre things happen. The times that I am talking about are not isolated to surgery. They are a part of everyday life. Call them kismet, fate, or destiny. But when bizarre things happen in surgery, there seems to be a heightened tone to them.

This incident happened early in my career. I was working for a large medical corporation selling surgical disposables. I started a small evaluation. It would last for one week, as most small OR evaluations do.

I was in the hospital OR dressed in surgical attire. I looked over the surgery schedule board. I targeted a procedure with a surgeon whom I had not met or worked with in any cases. The surgeon was a gynecologist. The procedure was scheduled to be a diagnostic vaginal procedure. I say scheduled to be. Often when you go into a procedure it turns out to be much more involved than it is scheduled to be. And it could evolve into a laparoscopic or open procedure that may last for hours.

A diagnostic procedure and other smaller procedures are mistakenly referred to as minor procedures or minor surgery. However, I have a different view of minor surgery. There is no such thing. Surgery that is performed on someone else is minor surgery. Any type of procedure that is performed on you is major.

I introduced myself to the surgeon at the scrub sink while he was prepping his hands. I asked him about the ensuing procedure. Showing interest in what a surgeon does helps to establish rapport and a relationship. Knowing what the procedure is and being able to talk medical terminology will further the trust that the surgeon needs to have in you for credibility. The doctor said that this woman came to him complaining of pain, a foul odor, and a darkened vaginal discharge. He had a medical history with her that went back a few years. She received a total hysterectomy from him. That day, he was going to scope her and find the cause of her current problems.

After scrubbing, we entered the OR to start the

procedure. The mood was light and friendly. Remember, this was just a diagnostic procedure. The patient was prepped and lying on her back with her legs and feet in stirrups. This is called the lithotomy position. A hysteroscope would be inserted into her vagina. A hysteroscope is a small, thin scope that is used to do a hysteroscopy. That procedure involves inserting the scope into the vagina, through the cervix and into the uterus. This allows the surgeon to view the uterus. Since this patient had a hysterectomy several years prior to that, he would only be viewing the vaginal canal.

Once the scope was inside the vagina, the surgeon began looking through the lens of the scope to inspect and discern what was causing her foul odor and dark discharge. Within less than a minute, he said, "Oh, my God, what is that?" He told the scrub nurse to hand him a pair of long sponge forceps. Still looking through the scope, he placed the forceps into the woman's vagina, clamped the tines together, and withdrew the instrument. Inside the instrument was a circular formation that had tentacle-like extensions on it. It was covered with a dark liquid. The smell in the room became overpowering. It smelled like necrotic tissue and pseudomonas. Pseudomonas are an infectious bacteria that may cause serious medical or surgical complications. Everyone in the room was gagging. The circulating nurse began spraying aerosols and offering liquid pine scent to place on the surgical mask to cover the stench.

The surgeon placed the object in a specimen cup and

took it to the back table to analyze. He said that he had never seen anything like it. He immediately called for the room to be quarantined. Nobody was to enter or leave until this object was sent to pathology and a report was returned. The circulator called for pathology to get the specimen. Meanwhile, we stood there with this sickening smell in the room.

Obviously, there was talk about the foreign object. The surgeon was really confused. He said that it was not a tumor, cyst, or growth of any kind. I asked him how long he thought that it had been inside her. He said that he did not know. But it had been there long enough to create an infection.

Fifteen minutes later (which seemed like hours), a pathology report came back over the intercom. The object in question was officially diagnosed as a French tickler. There was immediate laughter in the room. The tense situation had been defused by an erotic sex toy. The surgeon was laughing, smiling under his mask, and shaking his head. He said, "Like hell that woman did not know the cause of the smell. Her husband or boyfriend left it there."

After the procedure, I went to the nurse's lounge to get a cup of coffee. That procedure was the talk of the OR. It made for quite a few jokes and a day's worth of laughter.

It has been over thirty years since I was involved in that procedure. But when I think back on that smell, I still get a lump in my throat.

God Bless Those Who Save

We all know that with life comes death. It is a stark reality that we do not like to think about or dwell upon. The thought of our own mortality is enough to make us switch gears and think about the weather or if the home team is winning.

I believe in a natural right of passage in this life. That passage involves being born and reared by our parents. They take loving care of us as children. As we grow, our parents educate, guide, and instruct us. They teach us about life through their experienced eyes. As our parents grow older, there comes a time when the roles reverse—when the children take the role of parents and care for them until their time of eternal rest. That is the way that it should be. Children are supposed to bury their parents. It is not supposed to happen the other way around.

Life does not always work the way that it should. Events happen that are unthinkable. One of those events is the loss of a child. My beautiful wife and I have five children. The thought of losing one of them is more than I could withstand. I do not know how parents muster the courage to face a tragic event of that magnitude.

A certain group of parents justly humble me. They are the group of parents who, in the midst of their suffering and the agony of losing a child, find the strength, courage, and love to donate their children's organs for transplant. They are amazing human beings and should be thanked and praised.

I awoke one Sunday morning in the early fall. I jumped out of bed earlier than usual. The weather was supposed to be gorgeous. It was a game day and the team was at home. My wife and I were going to make an afternoon of it somewhere. Eat lunch and watch the game. Both of us were excited.

I received a phone call at seven in the morning from the operating room of one of my hospitals. They were harvesting a liver from a child that had expired. The child's parents donated the liver for transplant. The OR team would be performing that liver transplant sometime in the early afternoon. They would need me at the hospital around one to assist with setting up and using my equipment.

My wife heard the phone ring and came to ask me who was calling so early. She could tell from the look on my face that the call was something serious. I explained the situation to her. I apologized to her for not being able to spend the day with her. She said that she understood and that I had to go. And she said not to worry about her. She had been through this before.

I told her that I could not wait until one. I was leaving right away. I wanted to make sure that the OR had everything needed for the surgery. That meant I needed to have enough supplies to do three surgeries. It is important to always have backup supplies. She said that she understood that, also.

As I drove to the hospital, I felt so many mixed emotions. A Sunday afternoon of fun was not important anymore. All I could think about was the pain felt by the family that had lost a child and the excitement felt by the family of a four-year-old boy who would have a chance to live. My stomach was turning.

I arrived at the hospital about eight o'clock. I checked in, changed into OR scrub attire, and proceeded to the transplant room to find the head nurse. The staff would already be getting the room ready. And I had my checklist to go through before the procedure.

The transplant team was delighted to see me there so early. I checked out my equipment and surgical instruments. Everything was ready to go. I told the head nurse that I would be available in the nurses' lounge if any staff members had never been in-serviced on my equipment. She said that there were a few. She would send them when they had time.

For the next few hours, nurses came in and out of the lounge. I had my equipment set up for demonstration. Several stopped to hear my in-service. For some, it was the first time that they had heard the presentation. For others, it was a welcome refresher just before the procedure. I still had several hours before the transplant. I was ready and eager for it to start.

Transplant teams are fascinating. Their work is special, and so are they. What they do is serious and difficult. The work leaves them physically and emotionally exhausted. These procedures take many hours to perform. And it is impossible to not become emotionally attached to their patients. That is especially true when the patient is a young child.

The hour had arrived. The team was checking supplies, opening instruments, and positioning equipment in the room. The transplant organ was being readied. The young boy would soon be brought into the room to begin a new life.

I waited outside the OR for the surgeon to arrive. I had never met her before. She was new to the hospital. But the staff had the most wonderful things to say about her. They said that she was the best surgeon. She was fast and deliberate—not a wasted motion. She was kind to the staff and humble. That is unusual for a surgeon of her prestige and stature. They are usually arrogant, demanding, and abrupt with the nurses.

A few moments later, the surgeon arrived. I introduced myself to her, and we exchanged pleasantries. She thanked me for taking time on a weekend to be there. She apologized for the short notice. But she said that she was sure that I knew how these things happen. I asked her if she was comfortable using my equipment. She said that she was. She had used it for years at another university hospital. That was a vast reassurance to me.

After scrubbing, we entered the OR. I viewed this small young man lying on the OR table. He was such a tiny figure to be having such a big procedure. But he probably had been through so much already in his life. This was the type of procedure that only adults should have to endure. This is not supposed to happen to such a young child.

The surgery began. I watched as the surgeon moved with ease and grace, thanking the scrub nurse every time she was handed an instrument. I could hear small conversation and knew that she was smiling with the nurses at the OR table. She had a calming manner. It really helped to lower the stress level.

For the next five to six hours, I watched and waited for a question about a necessary clinical effect or a request to change the settings on my machine. There was silence. That was a very good sign. In these situations, silence means that all is going well.

An hour later, the circulating nurse told me that I could go home. I had been there for about ten hours, but I had planned to be there for the duration of the surgery. She assured me that she knew how to operate my equipment. She had used it for many years. And she said that the procedure was almost over. I told her that I would only leave if she promised to call me when the procedure was over. I wanted to know how the little guy was doing. She said that she would call.

As I was leaving the room, the surgeon called to me and thanked me again for all of my help. I sheepishly said that I did nothing. I told her she was the one who deserved thanks. She said, "No. I am only an instrument that is guided by a higher being." That was amazingly honest humility from a tremendously gifted surgeon.

When I arrived home, I was emotionally drained. And I had done nothing. I could only envision how that transplant team would feel when they were finished with the procedure. They would be physically and emotionally spent. But they would have a sense of pride about what they had accomplished. Their efforts would give a child and his family a chance for a life of joy and happiness.

About an hour later, my cell phone rang. It was the circulating nurse from the hospital. She called to say that the surgery was over, and the young boy was responding well. She thanked me for being there to offer support.

I hung up my phone and wept. I wept tears of sadness for the young boy who died and for the parents who lost their child but still found the courage and love to donate his liver. And I wept tears of joy for the young boy and his family who were given the beautiful gift of life.

God bless those who save.

Chapter 8 Endnotes:

1. Debra Novak and Stacey Benson, "Understanding and Controlling the Hazards of Surgical Smoke," *Becker's ASC Review*, March 28, 2011, http://beckersasc.com/asc-accreditation-and-patient-safety/understanding-and-contro.

2. Kay Ball, "Megadyne Current. Surgical Smoke Evacuation: Are You Compliant?," Megadyne Current, accessed January 27, 2013, http://www.megadyne.com/current_article.php?id=4.

Chapter 9
In Conclusion

My Swan Song

My life in the operating room has been an incredible surgical journey. It is a journey that has left me cynical of the established medical system in the United States. I have many recollections about my life in the operating room. Those recollections are a striking mixture. They transcend every imaginable emotion and feeling, and are as true as life can be. Unfortunately, as we all know, life can truly be a four-letter word.

Through my many years of working on the "inside," I have a keen understanding of the real surgical world. That world is ethically, morally, and economically in disarray. It no longer exists solely for the purpose of helping humanity and of being a welcome source of comfort for those who are in need. It has succumbed to the same greed and self-interests that underscore other business industries.

I believe corrections are needed in the way that health

care is perceived, conducted, and administered. I say this believing that there is a way to be compassionate toward the mission and successful in the business aspect. However, this would require a philosophical change. It would necessitate that those involved in the health-care industry not use it for a cash cow.

Current estimates are that over 25 percent of the yearly federal budget is spent on health care. It continues to increase as a percentage of the federal budget every year. I am convinced that if American health care is not modified and reversed, it will erode our basic economic system.

The health-care system in the United States is the finest in the world. In spite of obvious shortcomings, I would never consider being treated for any surgical diagnosis in any other country in the world. American surgical science is medical knowledge at its best.

There are many true caregivers in the surgical field. By doing your research, you will find a surgeon who cares about you and your medical condition. You will also find peace of mind knowing that you have made an educated and informed decision about the treatment path that you follow.

Working in the surgical world has left a mental mark on me that I will always remember. I leave it with a sense of comfort, satisfaction, and pride. It has provided my family and me a wonderful life. It has given me volumes of treasured memories. Most of the memories bring a warm smile to my face. Often, a pleasant memory will bring a sudden outburst of laughter. Other memories are not so pleasant and are sometimes painful. But such is life. You learn and move forward with eager anticipation of what the future will bring.

I wish you happiness and well-being.